# The Maternity Labyrinth

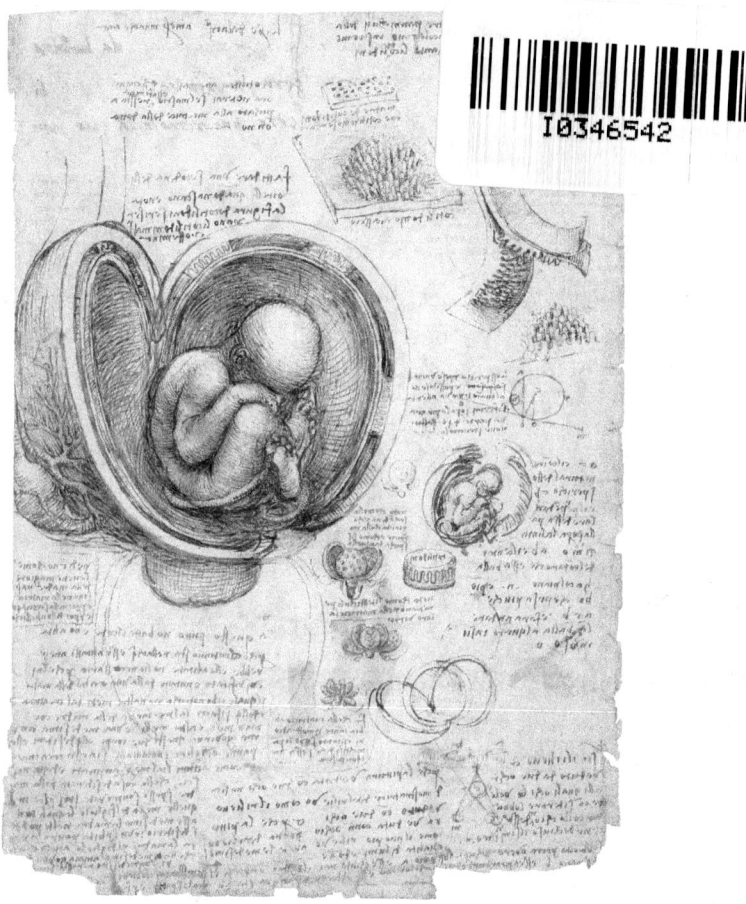

*Ariel Balter*

Plain View Press
P.O. 42255
Austin, TX 78704

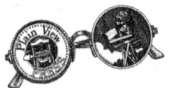

plainviewpress.net
sb@plainviewpress.net
512-441-2452

Copyright © 2010 Ariel Balter. All rights reserved under International and Pan-American Copyright Conventions. No part of this book may be reproduced or distributed in any form or by any means, or stored in a data base or retrieval system, without written permission from the author. All rights, including electronic, are reserved by the author and her publisher.

ISBN: 978-1-935514-54-1
Library of Congress Number: 2010928500

Cover art: *Leonardo da Vinci*. The Royal Collection copyright 2009,
        Her Majesty Queen Elizabeth II
Cover design by Susan Bright

## Acknowledgements

I'd like to thank Jayne Benjulian, Anne Detmer, Isabel Duffy, Alexandra Enders, Michael Fleming, Sarah Manyika, and Angela Sowa for sharing their wisdom and for their advice and assistance.

*Dedicated To Anna*

## Introduction

People rarely discuss pregnancy problems, infertility, in vitro fertilization, and miscarriages in public. Even though fifteen to twenty percent of pregnancies end in miscarriages, about ten percent of American couples of childbearing age have difficulty conceiving, more than 70,000 babies have been born in the United States using assisted reproductive technologies (ART), including 45,000 born as a result of in vitro fertilization (IVF), one in five pregnant women are prescribed bed rest for some period of their pregnancies, and eight to ten percent of births in the U.S. are pre-term, few seem to talk about their experiences in public, which is really quite odd considering that women make up about half the population and often have husbands or partners who are affected by these losses and difficulties. Is it simply the kind of topic that one does not discuss in mixed company, like menstruation, or is it too depressing to talk about at a dinner party, like mentioning a relative who has cancer? Why is the topic taboo despite its relevance to so many people?

Few people have qualms about discussing the achievements and talents of their own children with anyone and asking complete strangers if they have children. Those are perfectly acceptable topics of conversation. So how should women who have had reproductive problems respond when asked if they have children? What should a woman who barely has the energy to attend a social event because she has had multiple miscarriages or been on bed rest, or undergone years of fertility treatments say when asked if she has kids and, as a follow up question, what she does? It is certainly no surprise that some women would rather not discuss their experiences because they are too painful. Others may be ashamed that their bodies have failed them in the reproductive realm and that they are therefore deficient as women. They have good reasons to feel as they do. It's not simply that people don't want to hear about other people's problems. Instead, fertility and reproduction are, on some level, fundamental to who we are as human beings. They are the source of our existence, the perpetuation of our genes, our femininity or masculinity, and our own immortality. Thus failure in that domain signifies a particularly deep-seated inadequacy. Reproducing is something that most of us assume we can do successfully, like breathing and seeing. For most people, it comes as a shock when, during their childbearing years, they discover that they are unable to conceive or sustain a pregnancy. And because the subject is so fraught, compounded by the fact that science has no perfect remedies for infertility, it is no wonder that there is so much silence and unease about conception and pregnancy problems.

Given the prevalence of the issue, it is time that people were informed and talk about it. Women who conceive easily and breeze through their pregnancies and deliveries might think twice before assuming that such fortune applies to everyone. Conceiving and having a baby naturally do not require talent or brilliance, mostly luck. Judgments about who should have children and how they should have children are deeply unfair, particularly by those who have lost nothing and experienced no failures. In this day and age there are numerous ways to have a baby, including, adoption, IVF and other assisted reproductive technologies, surrogacy, egg and sperm donation, and some combination of the above. Intended parents have a right to choose which method is most appropriate for them based on their medical, financial, psychological, political, and moral positions. Nor should they be judged, particularly by those who can have children or who simply don't want children. People who adopt or undergo IVF or use a surrogate should be treated with the same, if not more, sympathy, kindness, and respect as those who have problem-free pregnancies, and they should feel proud to boast of their adopted or sperm-donor babies.

When asked, as I often was and still am, whether I have children, I stiffly responded, "no" and hoped the topic would change before the awkward silence and the follow-up question, "What do you do?," to which I more clumsily replied with some vague references to being a former teacher, who is now editing , tutoring, or writing. If pressed about what I write, I usually referred to something academic I've worked on and avoided mentioning this: my book about my own experiences with failed pregnancies, IVF, surrogacy, and seemingly endless loss and disappointment. So what have I been doing for the past few years besides writing, editing, and tutoring? I very well may have set a record for the longest human gestational period. I've been pregnant twice, on bed rest for a few months, gone into pre-term labor twice, lost two babies, undergone six rounds of IVF with two different surrogates, visited more doctors, hospitals, and fertility clinics than I can stand to remember, and tried to maintain my sanity and make some sense of all this.

Before I first went into labor, at the age of thirty-seven, I had never been a patient in a hospital and was fit and healthy. I had a basic trust in the competence of my doctors and in twenty-first century medicine. I assumed that most women who are generally healthy, fertile, get good pre-natal care, and take care of themselves will have successful pregnancies, or in the worst case, need medical intervention that will help them to have live, healthy babies. Evidently, I had idealized the powers of modern obstetrics and was unaware of the myriad complications and unknowns that are involved in human reproduction. Perhaps the reason I had heard so few stories about tragic pregnancies is because I had never been pregnant before or had serious health problems. Women generally share their reproductive misfortunes with others who have experienced them or their doctors. Otherwise, they keep quiet.

My story is about what not to expect when you're expecting. It is about how to cope with disbelief, disappointment, and grief. It is about the numerous possibilities that exist in reproductive technologies. There are many options out there for people who want children but cannot have them without some extra effort and help. For many, nowadays, the process of having a baby is nothing like it was in our mothers' time, but the end result, we hope, is pretty much the same. Although my story does have a happy ending, it is not a fairy tale or even a pep talk for those struggling with reproductive problems. In fact, one of the pitfalls of undergoing years of fertility treatments is that the process itself may become all-consuming and almost an end in and of itself, and it sometimes fails to provide the desired results; specifically, ARTs do not always work. Since my initial conception, the struggle to have a baby lasted over five years. I suppose you could say that, in my case, perseverance paid off. One friend who had had various fertility problems assured me that I would forget all of my travails as soon as I had a baby. Perhaps I will no longer dwell on my losses and disappointments and the process of getting a baby and instead, focus on the joys of motherhood and development of my child, but I certainly will not forget nor romanticize my experiences, nor will I ever be the same person I was five years ago. I can now say that my hard work was worth it, but my baby came at a very dear price.

# Chapter 1

Like many women who want kids and marry in their mid thirties, I wasted no time in trying to get pregnant. I even visited the gynecologist and began taking prenatal vitamins a few months before trying to get pregnant. Pretty much as soon as I was married, my husband Roger and I started trying, since we assumed that I had only a few fertile years left and was unlikely to get pregnant easily. Much to my astonishment, I became pregnant after only two months, despite paying little attention to ovulation cycles. When I told my husband, he looked at me in utter disbelief doubting the accuracy of the "99% accurate" test and my sanity. Quickly enough, the signs of pregnancy such as nausea, ravenous appetite, crankiness, swollen breasts and abdomen arrived to erase any doubts we were harboring.

Although I had a capable doctor, good health insurance and did not belong to a large HMO, my obstetrician in northern California would not see me for my first check up until I was at least ten weeks along. So I relied on information from *What to Expect When You're Expecting* and other maternity manuals to help me monitor the state of my own pregnancy. At about the ninth week, I started spotting and called the doctor's office. After leaving three unreturned messages, I called again, demanding, at least speak, to speak to a nurse. When I told her my symptoms, she replied in an annoyed, you're-wasting-my-time tone, that I was probably miscarrying and that I should just relax and put my feet up. There was nothing she or anyone else could do about it. I promptly found another doctor in private practice and was seen immediately. It turns out that I was not having a miscarriage and that the baby had a strong heart beat. All seemed well with the pregnancy.

Since I was over thirty-five and stood a fair chance of miscarrying, we decided not to tell anyone that I was pregnant until I had gotten through the first trimester and then inform only immediate family and close friends until after we found out the results of amniocentesis. So I just hoped that none of my colleagues at work noticed as I gained weight, wore loose fitting shirts, quit drinking coffee, visited the ladies room frequently, and spent a good bit of the day snacking. I felt a contradictory mix of emotions about my pregnancy: on the one hand, I was self-satisfied and almost cocky that I had gotten pregnant so easily and had made it through the first trimester. But I also worried that we'd find out our baby had Down's or some other serious genetic disorder and felt that I couldn't feel secure about the pregnancy until after all tests proved that baby and I were fine.

At around the seventeenth week of pregnancy I had amniocentesis. Prior to the procedure Roger and I were required to suffer through a genetic counseling session in which we were bombarded with statistics and lists of every possible genetic abnormality. Needless to say, after this session, and immediately prior to the test, we were convinced that our baby couldn't possibly be born without some sort of horrible genetic defect. At least I had already been screened for cystic fibrosis and Tay Sachs, so that we could probably rule out those two diseases. The amniocentesis was performed by a highly-recommended and sought-after doctor, Dr. C., who presumably had the finest track record in the San Francisco Bay area for fewest screw-ups of the procedure. He also had one of the poorest bedside manners I'd ever encountered. During the procedure he managed to offend everyone in the room by making redneck jokes about Oklahomans (my husband is from Oklahoma), racist jokes about Hispanic immigrant students who don't speak English (the nurse was Hispanic), and a crack about the New York City school population (I had been a teacher in a New York City public school). I suppose that Dr. C.'s comments distracted me from paying attention to the long needle in my abdomen. Perhaps that's what made him such a clever doctor.

About a week later we found out that we were having a perfectly healthy baby girl. Secure in the knowledge that the baby was fine, we proceeded to tell people about our exciting news, pick out baby names, and make plans. Since the baby was due in August and I was a teacher, I asked for a year leave so that I could spend time with our child. My comfort with the health of the pregnancy and baby improved as the weeks passed, especially after week twenty and the level-two ultrasound. Once again, everything seemed normal; her heart and all her other little organs, her spine and long fingers and toes looked perfect. We even had a small photo collection to show off our little fetus. She was an active baby who kicked often and seemed to flip around a lot in the womb, so we nicknamed her Jazzy B. At this point in my pregnancy, the glorious second trimester, I felt great—energetic, upbeat, hungry, and optimistic. I was following in the footsteps of my mother who had three easy, problem-free pregnancies.

One Monday night, in the middle of the twenty-fourth week I was lounging in bed, reading a novel, and generally feeling fine. I got up to use the bathroom and before flushing the toilet, noticed a bloody, mucousy clot in the water. I was alarmed but tried to convince myself that this might not be a serious problem. I calmly and dutifully consulted my various pregnancy guides. As I was sitting in bed poring through the books, I started having cramps. They must be Braxton-Hicks contractions, I told myself, since it was approximately the right time for those to begin. None of the books mentioned anything about bloody clots this far along in a pregnancy. I was certain I wasn't miscarrying since I was well past the first trimester. I was even weeks beyond the late miscarriage stage. Most of the pregnancy guides are organized by trimester, and there was simply no information about my symptoms in the second trimester chapters. There were some highlighted boxed off sections that warned women to call their doctors if they experienced bleeding at any time, but I wasn't even bleeding continuously. I told my sleeping husband about my symptoms and he suggested I call the obstetrician, Dr. M. Not wanting to pester her late at night and convincing myself that nothing could be terribly wrong since all tests, even very recent tests, proved that the pregnancy was healthy, I waited and fretted. After a few hours of consistent cramping, followed by increasing frequency and duration of contractions, though no further bleeding, I called the doctor who told me to go to the labor and delivery ward of the hospital where she would meet me. She later admitted that she almost hesitated to send me to the hospital since I sounded so calm and cool. So Roger and I got dressed and went off to the hospital in the dead of night. I didn't even pack a bag. I assumed I'd be home later that day. If modern medicine had the tools to see the four chambers of a fetus's heart, it could certainly stop some contractions. After all, my water hadn't even broken.

After arriving at the hospital and filling out various forms, we were ushered in to a labor and delivery room where I changed into a hospital gown and was hooked up to numerous monitors. I was certainly having contractions—painful, vigorous, frequent ones, but the baby still maintained a strong heartbeat and seemed okay. Since it was approaching dawn and the beginning of my work day I asked the nurse if I could use the phone to call in sick. Months later, the headmaster's assistant who listened to my voice mail told me how stunned she was by my nonchalant message saying that I wouldn't be in that Tuesday since I was in the hospital. I was still convinced that whatever was wrong could be fixed and, at the very worst, I'd be sent home to rest for a few days.

The labor and delivery nurse called my doctor, who was on her way to the hospital, and was directed to examine me. My cervix was significantly dilated; the nurse kept telling my doctor that she felt a big bag of water and was hesitant to continue examining me in case she broke the water sac. At this point I was beginning to realize that perhaps all was not so well. By the time Dr. M. arrived, I was fully dilated and having painful, body-wrenching contractions to the point of nauseating me. My doctor examined me and announced that she would have to do an emergency C-section since the baby was breach and she would never survive a vaginal delivery. I don't remember if I was numb, stunned, or still in a state of utter disbelief, but I hardly reacted other than assenting and thinking that a twenty-four and a half week old baby couldn't possibly survive.

Moments later the anesthesiologist and various other nurses and interns arrived. Doubled over in pain and feeling that I would throw up any second, I was rolled to my side and given a spinal as a nurse held a vomit bin by my mouth. I distinctly remember thinking that it would be just fine by me if I died at that moment. I simply wanted the pain to stop. The next thing I knew, my lower half was numb, the pain had disappeared, and my husband was putting on hospital scrubs and shoe protectors as the nurses were positioning a screen to prevent us from seeing my abdomen sliced open. Roger was directed to stand by my shoulder and avoid looking past the screen. He took hold of my hand and didn't let go during the entire procedure. In what seemed to be a very short time and a mere exchange of a few directions by the doctor (remember, I could feel or see nothing), out came a crying, kicking baby girl. Trying to be optimistic despite what we all knew was a poor prognosis, Dr. M. wearily declared, "It's a good sign that she's crying." The baby was promptly whisked off to the Neonatal Intensive Care Unit (NICU). We hardly got to lay eyes on her immediately after she was born; I was wheeled away to the recovery room.

Still feeling completely dazed but evidently recovered enough to be assaulted with more unwelcome news, I was wheeled down, accompanied by Roger, to the Neonatal Intensive Care Unit to consult with more doctors and see our baby. We were greeted, if you can call it a greeting, by the NICU attending physician whose first words to us were not hello or some standard comforting, I care phrase, but, "Babies born at twenty-four weeks have a fifty-fifty chance of survival." He continued that those who live are often blind, deaf, mentally retarded, have cerebral palsy and serious lung problems. Apparently our daughter was doing better than expected. She had no blood on the brain (a good sign), but her lungs were not well developed, which is usually the biggest problem for preemies. Our baby was likely to remain in the NICU for many months before she'd be well enough to come home with us-- that is if she got well. Roger was crying as I remained stone faced. I had yet to have much of a reaction to anything that had happened. The NICU looked like a scene from a science fiction movie. There were rows of plastic cribs or encasements that contained tiny, sickly looking babies who had numerous wires and tubes providing them with fluids, oxygen, and connections to monitors. One doctor seemed to be performing surgery on a baby in a crib a few feet away from us. Although we were assured that this was one of the most advanced NICUs in the country and that despite appearances, the newborns were not in pain, it looked to me like the babies were being tortured. There was nothing cozy or comforting about the Unit. My first reaction upon seeing our baby daughter was not one of warm maternal love. I may have even flinched. She weighed one pound, seven ounces. She was small and skinny and her skin was red and flaky. She looked a bit like an alien and nothing like the chubby-cheeked, fleshy, holdable babies I'd seen before. I was also scared to touch her because she was so tiny and frail and hooked up to so many machines. The nurse told us we could touch her hands or feet, which is what made me crack. Her hands and feet were miniature replicas of my own; she had my long skinny fingers and extra long second toes. The doctors and nurses proceeded to bombard us with information about preemies and told us that we could visit our baby whenever we wanted and they would update us regularly about her health. I was then taken upstairs to my hospital room.

Perhaps I should mention that, with the exception of my own birth, I had never been a patient in a hospital before. I had hardly even visited anyone else staying in a hospital. My family and friends tended to be a pretty healthy lot, and my friends who had babies were usually in and out of the hospital in a day or two, so most of my experiences visiting new moms and babies involved seeing normally dressed and bathed people sitting comfortably at home. The disinfectant-smelling hospital room, the plastic mattress pads, and the various machines and contraptions made me feel as if I were in a TV hospital drama. My brothers and I were fairly healthy children and my mother is not one to fuss about or reward sickness. If anything, we were raised to believe that we were somehow immune to serious illness or invincible. As far as anyone knew at that point, there was no reason why I had gone into premature labor. All lab results of tests for infection were negative. I did not have high blood pressure or gestational diabetes. I didn't smoke or use drugs. Failing to carry a baby to term and having a C-section were simply things that I believed couldn't happen to me and for which there were no good explanations. I hardly ever missed work or school because of illness. How could I not do what most women, even unhealthy women, seemingly accomplish so easily?

Once established in my room, which involved maneuvering me into bed after having had a C-section, reattaching IV needles, blood tests, and various other unpleasant procedures, Roger and I had a chance to be alone and try to process what happened. We were attempting to be optimistic about our baby's prognosis, but I think that we both knew that whether she lived or died, the outcome would be difficult. No sooner were we settled, then we were interrupted by a pushy, preposterously bubbly woman who began to lecture me about the importance of breastfeeding my baby. When I tried to explain, calmly, even though I felt like punching her, that our baby couldn't breastfeed because she was in the NICU, the woman insisted that it was all the more reason to nurse. She told me that she would arrange for a breast pump to be delivered to my room. My milk could be frozen and when the baby was well enough, she could have my milk which was much healthier than formula and would help mother and daughter bond. All I kept thinking was, couldn't we wait just a bit to see if our baby even survives. Sure enough, later that day a machine, which seemed to me like a miniature version of one used for milking cows, was delivered to my room. What can I say. There isn't much dignity in flinching in pain from an abdominal incision, wearing a hospital gown that leaves you half exposed, and trying to pump milk using a rather ungainly contraption when you think it's pretty pointless anyway.

Our next challenge was calling family and friends. We basically called immediate family and our closest friends and let them spread the word. Roger would start crying as he explained what happened, but I persisted in mechanically describing the situation and prognosis. I still hadn't shed a tear. We decided that local friends were welcome to visit us in the hospital since we'd be there for four days, but our parents who lived out of town shouldn't visit until at least a few days after we were home. The phone rang non-stop, and we continued to update everyone. We ourselves received periodic updates from NICU doctors about the health of our daughter. As the hours and days progressed her health deteriorated. In short, her lungs were not sufficiently developed, which led to a series of other serious problems. Throughout our stay at the hospital the doctors tried a variety of procedures to improve her lung function. On one visit to see our baby in the NICU and discuss her condition with the doctor we were interrupted, again, by the breast feeding advocate/cult member, who started to give her stump speech about the benefits of nursing. I don't remember who told her that this was not the right time for her oration, but it took a few cutting looks and remarks before she got the hint. The doctor's update made clear that it was unlikely we would need my breast milk.

Our situation finally became real to me the first night I slept at the hospital. I'm a very light sleeper under the best of circumstances, so I obviously couldn't sleep much in the noisy hospital in an uncomfortable bed and in pain from a C-section. Some time in the middle of the night when I wasn't being deliberately woken up by a nurse checking my blood pressure, I just started sobbing. Roger, who was permitted to stay in my room, was snoring away on the sleeper chair. Throughout our entire ordeal Roger was kind, supportive, steady, and comforting. If I were forced to come up with anything positive about our experience it would be that it brought us closer together and made me appreciate Roger even more than I already had. But that night, utterly exhausted, he slept soundly while I wept.

Among the many visitors including nurses, our doctor, social workers, and friends was a nurse or aide who requested that we fill out the form for a birth certificate which required the baby's name. How do you choose a name for a baby who is likely to die in a few days? Do you pick your favorite name, second favorite, a name that denotes grief or illness or doom? We delayed filling out the forms, despite frequent reminders by the staff, until it became apparent that we would also have to fill out a death certificate. It is necessary to have a birth certificate in order to have a legitimate death certificate. So we named her Emily, our favorite name, and it didn't keep her alive.

In the middle of the third night in the hospital, we received a call from a doctor in the NICU who informed us that Emily's health was deteriorating rapidly. Their last effort to improve her breathing had failed and there was now evidence that there was significant bleeding in her brain. They wanted to know what Roger and I wanted to do. Should Emily be taken off life support? Did we want to go to the NICU to see her before she died? They told us that they didn't think she had long to live. After discussing our options, which we determined weren't really options, we decided to have the life support removed. She couldn't breath on her own and would never have functioning lungs. The blood on her brain had probably already caused extensive brain damage. The doctors said that she wouldn't survive long while hooked up to the machines anyway. We concluded that there was no reason to prolong the agony and the inevitable. It was also unbearable to see such a small baby seemingly held together with tubes, needle, and tape. Roger and I informed the NICU doctor of our decision and went to visit Emily for the last time.

When we got to the NICU we were taken to a private room and told that Emily would be brought to us shortly. The room seemed reserved for grieving families and as a place to say good bye to their babies. We were also asked if we wanted a member of the clergy. I didn't, but Roger did. The idea of a stranger intruding on us and trying to comfort us with some prayer I'd heard hundreds of times was immensely unappealing to me. I was tired of talking to social workers and nurses and wanted to be with people I knew and loved or be left alone. I am also not particularly religious or big on praying. Roger liked the idea of saying goodbye in a more formal way and felt that a clergyman would be comforting. So, I acquiesced and the hospital chaplain on duty was summoned.

Given the location of the hospital, Silicon Valley, California, and the population using the hospital, largely white, Asian, and Hispanic, one would expect the hospital chaplain to be mainstream Protestant, Catholic, or Jewish, and white, Asian or Hispanic. But much to our amazement, in walked a snappily dressed African American Baptist minister. He was wearing a charcoal pinstriped zoot suit with a bright red shirt and a shiny, wildly patterned tie. His shoes were either black and white, or he was wearing spats; I couldn't get a good enough look without staring rudely. He introduced himself and asked us about our religions and what we wanted him to say. I was raised Jewish and Roger, Episcopalian. I made it clear that I wanted no references to Jesus and that a reading from the Old Testament was probably best. He assured us, perhaps detecting our astonishment or skepticism, that he could accommodate us and suggested reading the 23$^{rd}$ Psalm. Roger was pleased with that decision and I assented figuring it was innocuous enough; at that point I'd agree to anything that didn't involve getting on my knees, singing, and praising Jesus.

While we were chatting, a nurse and doctor brought in Emily, who was wrapped in a hospital blanket. She was still alive but fading. I was asked if I wanted to hold her. I honestly didn't because I was frightened and did not want to get attached to a dying baby or enfold a dead baby in my arms. But what could I say. Who would understand that? I assumed that saying no would be misinterpreted. Clearly, some psychologist or social worker had recommended this farewell ritual and I was supposed to obey despite the fact that I knew it would hurt more than help. So I nodded yes, and the nurse placed Emily in my arms. She was barely breathing, had poor coloring, and was quite still. For weeks after that I had horrible, wake-up-in-a sweat nightmares about holding a dead baby. Everyone, Roger, the minister, the NICU nurse and doctor then knelt in a circle and held hands. I was exempt from the prayer circle since I was holding Emily and couldn't kneel because of the C-section. I avoided catching Roger's eye because I didn't want to start laughing. I generally don't find religious ritual comforting, and this little gathering was absurd. Then we had a moment of silence. The doctor was crying. I was stunned. The scene was both terribly sad and utterly comical. What on earth were I, a Jewish New Yorker, and Roger, a reserved WASP, doing kneeling on the floor holding hands with a Baptist preacher when our baby was about to die? Mercifully, the service didn't last very long; the group dispersed, and Emily was whisked off by one of the nurses. A few hours later, we were informed that she had passed away.

After Emily died, we had to call family and friends again and make arrangements for a burial or cremation. We decided to bury her but have no funeral or memorial service. We couldn't bear arranging a funeral and sitting through a performance and ritual that seemed inappropriate for someone about whom there were few memories and who had hardly lived. The only memories to share and anecdotes to relate were private. Only I knew how her kicking felt when she was inside my womb; only Roger and I had seen her. What would we talk about in public? Her three awful days in the NICU at the hospital? Most of our family respected our decision. We agreed that my mother would visit a few days after we returned home. Roger's mother was told to come the following week, but she chose to ignore our wishes. Despite explaining clearly and rationally why we were not having a funeral, she persisted in calling my hospital room, repeatedly, only a few hours after our baby died, to lecture us on why we should have a funeral. "That's what's done," she said. "What will people think." She, who is not particularly religious, even had the gall to tell me, who was raised in a religious household, that religion is a comfort at times like this. I didn't find it the least bit comforting, just burdensome, maudlin, and insistent on its mind-numbing rhetoric. Why on earth would I want to affirm a faith in god now, of all times, and what good would it do me? In the end, my mother-in-law invited herself to what was supposed to be a private burial. She, like many others, decided she knew what was best. She also announced that she would be arriving the day after we returned home from the hospital.

The next morning, while packing up to leave, a nurse brought us a box of Emily's "effects." In it was a crocheted, pastel colored baby blanket, a card decorated with her footprints, a ceramic angel, and a hat. I'm not great at masking my feelings about people, so I'm not sure how I reacted. Perhaps I thanked her and maintained some composure until she left before I exploded. Her effects? What effects. She had no possessions. She was wearing a disposable diaper and lying in a sterile NICU crib on hospital sheets. The nurses must have had a room full of baby accoutrements that they gave to parents of NICU patients. I was horrified. I didn't want to remember the NICU, and I certainly didn't want a blanket that was never even used by Emily. Was this again something that psychologists suggested as a way to help remember or grieve for a baby? I took the card with her footprints of her feet which were so like my own and begged Roger to get rid of the rest of the items. I'm sure that the nurses meant well, but the angel and the unused blanket were silly and offensive to me.

Besides, when we arrived home, we were confronted by a house filled with Emily's effects, and those were only too real a reminder of what we had lost. My maternity clothes and pillows were all over our bedroom. We had bags full of baby gifts and hand-me-downs from friends and relatives. *What to Expect When You're Expecting* was still on my bedside table. The web site was still open on Roger's computer for the hospital tour and birthing classes in which we were planning to enroll the night I went into labor. And then there were countless bouquets of flowers and fruit baskets left on our front porch and many more that would continue to arrive for the next few days. Roger spent a good part of the day calling morticians and cemeteries to arrange for Emily's burial. Although it was an improvement over the hospital, home was no comfort or place to heal and forget. Everything in our house assaulted us with mementos of my pregnancy and Emily's death.

In the middle of our first night back at home I was awakened by a loud thud or crashing sound. Unable and uninspired to get up, I brushed it off as the usual noises of an old creaky house. When I went downstairs the next morning, I noticed a large bulge and crack on one wall of the living room. I figured that the long-standing hairline crack had simply expanded and I sighed, annoyed that we'd have to paint and plaster sooner rather than later. Also, Roger noticed that the front door and some of the closets seemed to have expanded overnight and weren't closing properly. Everything else appeared intact and functioned normally in the house, so we just went on with our day. Later that morning when I was about to get into the shower, I noticed that there was no hot water. Roger went down to the basement to check the water heater and sure enough solved the mystery. The entire basement was flooded because the bottom of the water heater had fallen out. Apparently, the flood of water and ensuing mud pit in our basement unsettled the foundation of the house causing various walls to bulge and crack. It was as if our home had gone into preterm labor as well. Later that day the plumbers came and replaced the water heater and drained the basement. After the walls and basement dried out a few weeks later the painters came to fix the house including the baby's room that we no longer needed. Unlike me, after a lot of mess and work, the house looked better than ever.

That day Roger's mother arrived to be unhelpful and to attend a burial to which she was not invited. Although she didn't stay with us, she demanded our time and attention. She doesn't cook well, won't drive anywhere but in her own town, and isn't strong enough to do any useful errands. Her visit required Roger to drive her around on pointless errands while I was left home alone, though remaining by myself was preferable to being lectured and interrogated by her. Besides I now had time to find something to read at Emily's burial. Despite spending many years in graduate school for a Ph.D. in English, I had a hard time finding an appropriate poem to read. None really fit; most mourning poems or elegies were about parents, spouses, or even older children. Anne Bradstreet wrote about losing a grandchild, but she was too religious for my taste. I, the religious cynic couldn't very well read a poem written by a Puritan. Besides, children died in childbirth often in those days. People had numerous children and usually lost some of them. It was expected. But this is the twenty-first century. Babies aren't supposed to die anymore.

The next day the three of us drove to the cemetery to bury Emily. We buried her in a lovely spot with a view of the Pacific Ocean and nearby mountains, but the children's section of the cemetery was horrifying. There were hundreds of tiny graves marked by small plaques many engraved with pictures of angels. Most of the graves were littered or decorated with stuffed animals, flowers, toys, and pinwheels. Even the graves of babies who had died many years ago were still adorned with children's goods. Clearly parents were still maintaining and visiting their children's burial plots. Surprisingly, there were quite a few parents and extended families standing by their lost ones' graves. I wondered how long one mourned a child who had hardly lived. I could hardly stand to visit the cemetery for the burial; how could these people build shrines and dwell on the loss of their children year after year? Perhaps they were the same people who wanted their baby's "effects." Did they find it comforting to visit the grave or purchase maudlin knickknacks like stuffed animals to remind them again and again that they had lost a child? I had no problem remembering. In fact, I could do nothing but replay, over and over again, every moment of my ordeal. I wanted my house and neighborhood to be free of baby and pregnancy reminders; I wanted to walk around happy and carefree without wincing at the sight of a pregnant woman; I wanted my pre-pregnancy, scar-free body back; I wanted my sore, engorged breasts to figure out that there was no baby to nurse; and most of all, I wanted a healthy, full-term baby. Reading a Bible passage and a few poems were egregious reminders for me. So we read psalm 23, again, and a poem by Thomas Hardy, and got back in the car and returned home to remember some more.

## Chapter 2

Presumably, now that the burial was completed, the visiting family members had returned home, and I was resting, the healing process could begin. A friend of mine who had had two C-sections warned me that it would take a good two weeks before I would stop wincing in pain every time I stood up or sat down. She was right. It also took at least one week from the time my milk came in for the engorgement to recede and for me to find it bearable to walk around without ice packs or cabbage leaves on my breasts. Given that I had undergone abdominal surgery, it would be some time before I could exercise again and regain any semblance of my pre-pregnancy figure. No doubt all of these physical discomforts afflict any woman who has just given birth via C-section, but instead of accepting that those were the costs of pregnancy and childbirth, I was resentful and angry. I felt that I had nothing to show for my pain and disfigurement and that I had a long ugly scar for nothing. Friends joked that at least I wasn't sleep deprived as most new mothers were, but I would gladly have traded places with a tired mother of a healthy newborn than felt exhausted and achy and childless.

Besides, who said that I wasn't sleep-deprived. For weeks I woke up every night numerous times because it hurt to turn from one side to the other. I also was awakened frequently by horrible nightmares involving dead babies and hospital intensive care units. I'd find myself drenched in sweat, my heart pounding, and unable to go back to sleep. The psychological part of the healing process took far longer than the physical side. To this day I think of myself as damaged and believe that I will never be the same person I was before I went into labor. I basically go about my business: I work, socialize with friends and family, run errands, and exercise, but I often feel somewhat disengaged. I simply don't see the world the way I once did. I have no faith that my body that had always been pretty strong, healthy, and athletic will function normally; I no longer trust in the miracles of modern medicine or that doctors do much more than educated guesswork; and I feel that there is absolutely no justice. Everything does not happen for a reason, and life is deeply unfair. I had always been a bit of a skeptic, but this experience brought me to a whole new level of cynicism.

About a week after I got home I had my first appointment with my obstetrician to remove stitches and check on my incision. Dr. M. seemed as interested in monitoring my mental state as my physical well-being. She still didn't know why I had gone into pre-term labor and recommended that I see a perinatologist or high-risk pregnancy doctor and gave me a referral. I had none of the traits (hypertension, obesity, diabetes, infection) or habits (cigarette smoking or drug use) that often trigger pre-term labor. She also quizzed me about my emotional state, asking if I was sleeping and eating normally or crying frequently and offered to give me a prescription for Prozac. I'm not terribly weepy by nature, so the fact that I wasn't crying regularly was no measure of my depression level. Too, since when do obstetrician/gynecologists prescribe anti-depressants? If I had agreed to take the drug, would she have monitored me for adverse reactions? Isn't it normal and healthy to grieve after losing a baby? Perhaps it would have been appropriate for her to intervene if I wasn't able to get out of bed two years later, but feeling blue two weeks after such a loss certainly doesn't warrant taking Prozac. I know that she meant well, was concerned about me, and probably felt terrible about what had happened, but I could accept being sad for a while.

Dr. M. also gave me some brochures for support groups and the name of a psychologist. The support groups seemed to be aimed more at women who had experienced miscarriages; the organizations also had such unfortunate names as "Helping Hands" or "Holding Hands" with fliers decorated with handprints that looked like they'd been designed by four-year olds doing arts and crafts in a pre-school program. The groups felt completely inappropriate for me. First of all, I had not had a miscarriage. Giving birth after twenty-four and a half weeks of pregnancy is not the same as miscarrying in the first trimester. Women who miscarry do not have C-sections and give birth to live babies. Although miscarrying is terribly sad and can be devastating to some women, it is fairly common and not unexpected, particularly in women over thirty-five. Going into labor when I did is quite uncommon, particularly given my general health, medical history, and normal pregnancy and baby; it was completely unexpected and, at that point, inexplicable. Second, group therapy is my idea of a bad dream or comedy act. Anyone who knows me well would laugh at the idea of me attending a rap session about miscarrying. I am not one to cry on other people's shoulders or discuss my mental state with perfect strangers. I was more than happy to talk to a competent psychologist or friends and family, but there was no way that I would hold hands with and weep and hug other miserable women whom I did not know.

Reading literature on grief was no help either. I didn't want to read about mourning and loss. Why would I want to wallow in my misery or someone else's? Also, most of the articles and books I read didn't quite apply. Unlike someone who loses a spouse, parent, or grown child, I didn't exactly lose someone who was a significant part of my life. I didn't know Emily or love her in the way one loves a growing, viable child. I was mourning the idea or hope or potential of Emily. I had lost optimism and faith in my body and in medicine. I felt hopeless and distrustful. Is that the same thing as traditional grief?

Soon after I returned home from my appointment with Dr. M., I decided to call the perinatologist she had recommended, Dr. D. I wanted to know why I had gone into early labor and if it was likely to happen again should I get pregnant in the future. I still very much wanted to have a child and felt that the only way to ameliorate my loss was to try again and have a successful pregnancy. Perhaps getting a logical explanation of what happened would restore a bit of trust in medicine and provide me, at the very least, with the illusion that I could have some element of control over my next pregnancy. Maybe there was some drug I could take or regimen I could follow that would enable me to carry to term. So I called the doctor's office to set up a consultation with him. I had been warned by my obstetrician that as the highly renowned and respected chief of his department Dr. D. would be very busy and hard to see despite her referral and my history. When I called to set up an appointment I was put on hold numerous times and transferred to different nurses and assistants until I was finally connected to his scheduling nurse who then gave me the third degree. While being interrogated about my pregnancy and medical history, I just snapped and began sobbing at which point his nurse toned down her questioning a bit and granted me an appointment date—three months from then. It seemed that getting a consultation with him was like interviewing for a job or applying to graduate school. Although in this case, the more deficient and impaired I was, the more likely I was to be accepted. Evidently I passed the test.

In the months preceding and waiting for what I hoped would be a revelatory medical consultation with an illustrious doctor, I began to resume my usual routines and returned to work. Innocuous tasks like walking to the post office, or visiting the dentist, the gym, and the supermarket were fraught with anxiety, discomfort, and awkward moments. It seemed that every block and every store were overrun with pregnant women or new mothers pushing strollers. Had there been a new baby boom in California, and specifically, in my neighborhood? The big, proud pregnant women confidently parading their large bellies bothered me the most. Although I knew logically that most women carry to term and can walk and even exercise all the way up to the day they deliver an eight-pound baby, I was still amazed and offended by them. I know I stared, hoping to glean some secret to their success, wondering how, when eight months pregnant, they carried groceries, rode bikes, and lifted toddlers with no ill consequences.

And how could they know what I was thinking as they smiled at me oblivious that their presence was an affront to me. It was surreal to spend many months feigning cheerfulness, or at least composure when I was all-consumed by thoughts of what had happened. I appeared to be relatively sane. I wasn't walking down the street and talking to myself or crying or gesticulating wildly. Perhaps I had a distracted or less than amicable look on my face but nothing that would indicate the depth of my sorrow or what I had only recently undergone. I also found it frustrating that Roger appeared to be recovering more easily than I. He's generally better at denial or compartmentalizing different facets of his life. Also, for men, losing a baby is not a visceral experience; they don't carry or deliver or nurse, and they undergo no physical pain or healing in relation to child bearing. Nevertheless, in imitation of Roger or just in an effort to maintain some semblance of normalcy and my previous self, I forced myself to take walks, run errands, see friends, go to movies—any form of distraction and routine. Maybe by playing the role of a happy, well-adjusted person I would become one again.

It did not help matters that my mother-in-law chose to be particularly sadistic during my "healing" period. One night, when Roger happened to be out of town she called. In the midst of her endless babbling and dispensing of unsolicited advice, she told me, "The only reason Roger married you was to have a baby. He really wants children." I don't remember how I responded to her other than cutting the phone call short and hanging up. The next day Roger informed me that his mother had called him after talking to me and confessed to saying something "bad" without specifying what.

I returned to work four weeks after giving birth despite my doctor's suggestion that I wait two more weeks. I felt relatively well physically and wouldn't need to do any heavy lifting at school, and I desperately needed a distraction. Sitting at home and stewing was not helping matters. Also, since Roger had already returned to work, I had no company during the day and noticed that being busy was helpful to him. For the most part, dealing with my colleagues at work wasn't too difficult. Everyone already knew what had happened, and I had already seen and talked to my closer work friends. Many of my colleagues had been bringing over meals and keeping me up to date about goings-on and school gossip. In general, the community was supportive and kind without being maudlin or prying. It's interesting what people whom you've known for a while will suddenly confide in you once you experience a loss. Three women I worked with, all with healthy, grown children, had babies who had been stillborn or died shortly after birth. You would never know it from talking to or interacting with them. They are all productive, pleasant people. Perhaps I wouldn't have to spend the rest of my life feeling like I was walking around with a dark cloud hovering over my head. Maybe, as they say, time heals all or most wounds. Or maybe they were faking it as I was, only they had had more time to polish their acts.

Seeing my teenage students again was harder. For starters, I had never told them that I was pregnant (it had been fairly obvious), so it would be strange to relate what had recently transpired. Also, being teenagers, most of them were quite self-absorbed, and my loss was so far outside the realm of their own experiences or concerns that I decided to just return to business as usual. There were books to read and discuss, papers to write, and finals to take. My students didn't need to know about my personal travails and I didn't feel like discussing them with kids. After all, I had returned to work so that I could think about something else. Again, I went through the motions and tried to seem enthusiastic and attentive. A year and a half later the head of school, who had been so accommodating, sent a rose bush after our loss, and acted deeply concerned for my well being, told me in an accusatory, chastising tone that I had seemed disengaged and wasn't interacting with students enough. "No shit," I thought. It was startling to me that he, who was a father and had exhibited moments of sensitivity, didn't get it. I was incapable of true engagement with that job and particularly since it involved dealing with children. Like the pregnant women who roamed my neighborhood, these kids were a reminder of what I couldn't have. Although it served as a distraction, to me, the school was also strongly linked to losing a baby. That's where I was employed when it happened and that's where I returned soon after. It took an extraordinary amount of effort to get up every morning and do my job competently. No one could force me and I couldn't force myself to become engaged and enthusiastic.

In some ways, the daily, casual encounters I had were far more distressing than dealing with people at work or friends and family. I frequently found myself having to explain to an embarrassed someone I hardly knew that I had lost a baby. Clerks at the dry cleaners or other stores I visited regularly would ask about the baby or my being pregnant, and I'd have to tell them that it was all over. The dentist and dental hygienist knew I had been pregnant because I couldn't have x-rays when I'd had my teeth cleaned a couple of months earlier. On my next visit I had to explain what had happened and was then forced into a long and painful conversation with the hygienist when she had me captive in the chair as she prepared to clean my teeth. Ironically, the gym, which I joined a few weeks after delivering so that I could get back into shape and feel better about myself, was probably the most stressful place to frequent. The majority of the gym goers were thirty-something year old women who were either pregnant or had young children. On my first day at the gym, I had to explain to the trainer who was helping me use the machines and develop a routine that I had recently had a C-section and wanted to strengthen my abdominal muscles. A few weeks later I ran into him and mentioned that I was going on a short vacation to which he replied, "Are you going with your husband and baby?" It certainly wasn't unreasonable for him to assume that I had a baby given that I had had a C-section. However, I then said something awful like, "There is no baby. She died," which was followed by his terribly awkward silence and embarrassed look. Since that day he has hardly said a word to me. A few months after Emily died we received Roger's alumni bulletin from engineering school. Sure enough, in the class notes section was a blurb on Roger that included information about his career and mention of his wife Ariel and daughter Emily. To this day we have no idea how they got such information. We certainly never updated the alumni office about anything other than a pregnancy. In addition to the usual proliferation and prominence of pregnant women, there were constant reminders like these that went on for many months.

Just as the school semester was ending, Roger had to fly to Paris for a few days for work and suggested I accompany him. Literally fleeing the country seemed like a great idea and the perfect form of distraction and escapism. While on the plane I made the mistake of reading an article in the the *New Yorker* by a man who was describing his and his wife's ordeal with in vitro fertilization (IVF) and travails of infertility and miscarriage. For some perverse reason I read the whole article despite finding the subject matter painful and feeling offended that a man could so light-heartedly describing his wife's experiences. Although their IVF procedure was finally successful, I vowed then and there that I would never undergo the procedure or have anything to do with a fertility doctor. The writer's description made the fertility business seem like a game and a lucrative enterprise that was interested in producing a pregnancy with little regard to cost for the woman; the smug writer/husband to me seemed guiltiest of abusing his wife and having the gall to write about it as if he had undergone the procedure. After calming down, I noticed that an old college acquaintance was sitting in the row in front of me. I managed to avoid her for most of the long flight specifically because I did not want to talk about what I'd been up to recently. As luck would have it, there was no avoiding each other when deplaning or waiting in line at passport control. So, once again, I had to at least allude to, some baby or pregnancy-related experience. Fortunately, the rest of the trip served as a wonderful diversion.

Not long after we returned from France we started receiving calls from the hospital that our insurance wouldn't cover certain costs and that we owed the hospital a great deal of money. These calls persisted despite the fact that our insurance was supposed to cover all hospital bills and that I had called the insurance company multiple times to straighten out a mistake that they had made. Although the insurance company had messed up, it was the hospital accounting department that showed a complete lack of sensitivity. It seems to me that harassing and threatening people who have recently lost a baby is bad policy. Although hospitals need to be paid whether or not they cure their patients, they could exercise more diplomacy particularly when dealing with families of those who were not saved.

Finally, after three long months the day of my appointment with the perinatologist arrived. His office had the misfortune of being located in the hospital in which Emily was born and died. I was shaking as I walked through the front doors and down the long corridor to his office. At least I didn't have to pass by the maternity ward or the NICU. After checking in I sat in a dingy waiting room for over an hour. The waiting area in this children's hospital was populated by pregnant women and parents with their sick young children waiting to be seen in another department. Clearly it never occurred to anyone that having women with high risk pregnancies share a waiting area with terribly ill children was not the brightest idea. Meanwhile, Roger, who had accompanied me hoping to join in the medical consultation, had to leave to catch a flight. He had falsely believed that an hour would be sufficient time for a doctor's appointment. When I was finally called in, I met with a Fellow in the high risk pregnancy department who interviewed me for about forty-five minutes and reviewed my medical records; she then left the room and me waiting some more until the expert, Dr. D., arrived.

Although I had enjoyed talking with the Fellow and she seemed perfectly competent, I was utterly exasperated and annoyed with waiting for the doctor. At last, Dr. D., accompanied by the Fellow entered. The doctor, who looked like a troll, brusquely introduced himself and began to question me further and review my situation. Although I had never had an abortion, my mother had never taken DES (Diethylstilbestrol to avoid miscarriage), and she had three normal pregnancies, he postulated that I have an incompetent cervix. An incompetent cervix, a bizarre term that could only have been coined by a man, is a weak cervix that opens prematurely and without labor or contractions during pregnancy. Labeling a cervix "incompetent" suggests a character flaw and fault on the part of the woman. Nevertheless, approximately one to two percent of women have incompetent cervixes and twenty to twenty-five percent of babies born in the second trimester are due to this. I had none of the typical attributes of someone with an incompetent cervix, and my carrying to twenty-four weeks was unusually long for such a condition, making the doctor less than certain about his diagnosis. It's also unclear what exactly prompts the cervix to dilate too early in the pregnancy. I explained to Dr. D. that I wanted a child and desired to know if there was a way I could carry to term. He recommended that should I become pregnant, I would need to get a cerclage (a surgical procedure in which the cervix is sewn shut) at about twelve to thirteen weeks along and then go on bed rest for the remainder of the pregnancy. The rationale behind bed rest is a bit murky. Although it may put less weight and strain on the cervix, it can also cause other health problems like poor circulation, blood clots, bed sores, and depression. Bed rest is a controversial and probably over-prescribed treatment, but it's often recommended because it tends to help more than hurt. He advised that I be monitored by a high risk pregnancy specialist and not my regular obstetrician. When I asked him about success rates with bed rest and cerclage he was non-committal. Approximately eighty-five percent of women who have a cerclage carry to term or close to term, but the numbers aren't that accurate partly because pregnant women are prescribed bed rest for a large variety of reasons and the statistics don't distinguish among the many reasons behind bed rest. Also, he couldn't know for certain if I even had an incompetent cervix since one needs to go into pre-term labor twice to prove it. My choices were to get pregnant and go about my business as if everything were fine and in the off chance that his diagnosis was wrong and the disaster of my first pregnancy was a mere fluke. Or, I could get a cerclage, perhaps needlessly and go on bed rest, or do just one of the above. I was determined to get pregnant and have a healthy, live baby. I felt that the only way to remedy or ameliorate my loss was to have another child, and I decided to do whatever was fairly reasonable and necessary to have a baby.

Since the perinatologist's recommendation seemed rather extreme to me I decided to seek out a second opinion. If I was going to have my cervix stitched shut and be on bed rest for six months I wanted to be certain that I was making the right decision. So I set up an appointment with another well-respected high-risk pregnancy doctor, Dr. O., in another university hospital in San Francisco. I was referred to this doctor through a friend who did research at that medical school and found out that the doctor had written a book on bed rest and avoiding pre-term labor. Although visiting her office did not quite feel like returning to the scene of the crime as it did in the previous hospital, it was still uncomfortable sitting in a waiting room populated exclusively by very pregnant women. No sooner than moments after being taken into the doctor's office, and explaining my situation, I was assaulted with Dr. O.'s assertion that "you realize that you can't replace the baby you lost." "No kidding," I thought looking irked. Was this some line that doctors learned during their psychiatric rotation? Did she think that I would name the second child Emily? I simply wanted a child and was well aware that I couldn't have the same one. Again, the medical doctor who was supposed to be discussing my cervix or some other part of my reproductive system decided to play psychiatrist. After merely glancing at my medical records, she too concluded that my cervix is incompetent and that if I got pregnant, I should have a cerclage and go on bed rest. Although she wasn't nearly as thorough as Dr. D., she did make the same diagnosis and recommendation. I guess I had my answer; if I wanted to stay pregnant for nine months I would undergo surgery and be confined to bed. It seemed rather Victorian to me, but if two experts came to the same conclusion, then who was I to question them.

## Chapter 3

A few months after we lost Emily and I was deemed fully recovered physically, we started trying to get me pregnant again. Becoming pregnant took on a kind of urgency. Roger and I deeply wanted a child, and I probably didn't have too many remaining fertile years. I also felt that I had something to prove or remedy, namely, carrying a baby to term. Since we felt pressed for time, we decided to approach the task more scientifically than we had in round one even though getting pregnant hadn't been a problem. So I purchased ovulation kits and paid attention to my cycles, took prenatal vitamins, and generally tried to lead a healthy lifestyle. Maintaining constant vigilance over when one has sex and whether one is pregnant or ovulating does little but cause added stress and anxiety. But after seven months, I found myself pregnant again. Perhaps I wasn't as fertile as I had been a year-and-a-half earlier, but with some effort and luck I managed to conceive a second time.

I was amazed that I had agreed to something that I would never have thought myself capable or willing to undertake—surgery and six months of bed rest without any guarantee, though good odds of having a baby. But I was on a mission and planned to arm myself with as much information, medical intervention, creature comforts, and help as I could to get me through the next nine months. The timing was perfect. The end of the first trimester, when I would undergo the cerclage and begin bed rest coincided with the end of the school year. By taking a year-long leave from work, I would have the time to recline horizontally for six months and get the added bonus of seven months at home with our new baby. So I made appointments with my obstetrician, Dr. M. and the high risk specialist, Dr. D. My regular obstetrician saw me immediately. The baby had a fine heartbeat, and the pregnancy seemed normal so far. The perinatologist wouldn't see me until I was at least ten weeks along. He wasn't particularly concerned with the first trimester and seemed to have the attitude that miscarriages couldn't really be prevented early on; let nature take its course. Dr. D. would intervene at around twelve weeks when he believed that he could thwart nature's ways.

My regular obstetrician, perinatologist, and I formed a sort of alliance in which I would be monitored by both of them. I would see Dr. M. every other week for regular checkups and blood tests and Dr. D. every two to three weeks for checkups, ultrasounds and any extraordinary procedures like the cerclage or serious problems that might arise. It was agreed that I would undergo CVS (chorionic villus sampling, a prenatal test that involves taking a tissue sample from outside the sac where the fetus develops) in the tenth or eleventh week and the cerclage at around the twelfth or thirteenth week. The perinatologist wanted to be certain that all was well with the baby before he sewed me up, and amniocentesis was performed too late in the pregnancy to obtain the information necessary to justify a cerclage. Also, I suspect that he didn't want anything to ruin his handiwork.

I spent the next few weeks putting my affairs in order for what felt to me was a six month long sentence under house arrest. I arranged the year leave from my job and stockpiled provisions and amusements for my period of confinement. Roger planned to go on a reduced schedule at work so that he wouldn't need to travel and could be home to prepare meals for me. An acquaintance of mine from graduate school had been put on bed rest twice because of an incompetent cervix and had two healthy children. I called her and got lots of advice and encouragement. Here was someone for whom this procedure worked and who chose to undergo it a second time. So I figured that despite its difficulty, it was bearable and evidently worthwhile. My friend's children were concrete evidence that this intervention could be effective. I was also seen by Dr. D. shortly before the CVS procedure. He confirmed that I was in fact pregnant and ready to be tested, stitched up, and confined to bed. Although the waiting area for his practice was as depressing and dingy as ever, at least the time spent waiting to see the perinatologist was within reason. Now that I was officially pregnant and officially his patient, I would be treated decently.

When I was around ten and a half weeks pregnant I underwent chorionic villus sampling to determine if the baby had any genetic diseases. This time the procedure was done at the hospital by another highly competent and even friendly doctor. In order to get to the room in which the procedure would be performed I had to walk past the NICU. Once again, I felt queasy retracing my steps in the hospital and knew that I'd be taking that route often, every time I came in for an ultrasound. Once again, Roger and I were tormented by the genetic counselors even though we had already been educated about genetic disorders before I had amniocentesis. The procedure itself, which entailed putting a tube through my cervix, was more unpleasant than amniocentesis, but went smoothly. A week later we found out, once again, that we were expecting a healthy baby girl. We were relieved but cautiously optimistic. I no longer had any illusions that getting through the first trimester and passing prenatal testing meant that I would carry to term and have a healthy baby. I had one week remaining before the cerclage and the temporary loss of my freedom.

On the appointed day, we returned to the hospital once again, specifically to the area near the labor and delivery department. After checking in and filling out lots of paperwork, I was prepped for surgery and taken into the operating room. Roger was spared watching this procedure. For the second time in my life I met with an anesthesiologist and was given a spinal. I remember being amused when he took my blood pressure and pulse and asked if I was a runner. I hadn't exercised at all since I found out I was pregnant; in fact, I had never been so sedentary in my entire life. So much for exercise and heart health, I thought. The procedure itself went well and I felt no pain, only a weird tugging sensation. When my cervix was properly sewn up, I was wheeled to a recovery room where Roger met me. The room was fairly small and had two beds separated by a curtain. Lying in the other bed was a woman who had just given birth and was being instructed on how to nurse her newborn. While I was recovering from the surgery and the anesthesia I had to listen to someone cooing over, nursing, and even picking a name for her baby. Clearly as much thought went into selecting recovery roommates as into designing a waiting area for the high risk pregnancy ward.

Here I was just beginning my long period of bed rest. We decided that I would confine myself to the sofa in the den, which was well situated next to a bathroom and the kitchen. When I asked what exactly I was permitted to do while on bed rest Dr. D. responded that I could get up to use the bathroom and I could walk around the house a few minutes a day. I could also shower quickly. Since our bedroom is on the second floor of our house, the doctor said that I could go upstairs at night to sleep and come downstairs in the morning. In general, his prescriptions were somewhat vague and unhelpful. I had to ask him particular questions about showering and driving because he did not provide me with concrete rules. Apparently, I could drive myself to doctor appointments since they were close by. It seems that he wanted me on my feet and sitting up as little as possible. The less weight on my cervix, the better. Everyone I've ever talked to who's been on bed rest was given different rules. Some people are forbidden to drive, others aren't. Some can't lift anything, not even a book or sandwich, and others can prepare meals for themselves. Some have to use bed pans while others can get up and use the bathroom like healthy mobile people. From what I could determine, I wasn't on the strictest form of bed rest, but I also wasn't on the most lenient.

The den was prepared for maximum comfort and convenience. In front of the sofa a small table was set up with my laptop. I had purchased many new books, joined Netflix and had a fine stash of DVDs. The phone, water and snacks were all within arm's reach. I had even ordered a bunch of DVDs and CDs and books to teach myself Spanish. Right before starting bed rest we signed up for a food home delivery service. We could order prepared meals online and have them delivered to the house once a week. Roger made breakfast for me and got lunch prepared before he left for work. He was usually home to warm up the catered dinners. The most I ever had to do was walk to the refrigerator and grab a snack or microwave something. We seemed to be making the best of a difficult situation.

Much to my surprise, the worst part of being on bed rest wasn't the boredom or loneliness, but the physical discomfort. Lying on one's sides and a bit on one's back for weeks on end is plain uncomfortable. I always seemed to have a stiff neck or shoulders. I was also antsy. I'm the type who is constantly moving; even when I'm sitting and reading or watching a movie, I tap my feet or drum my fingers or get up numerous times for pointless tasks. Staying horizontal and minimizing my movement was maddening. One friend who had had a difficult pregnancy, recommended a masseuse she had used who made house calls. The masseuse worked part-time at a hospital and was trained in pre-natal massage. I checked with my doctors who approved the idea. I figured she might help my stiff neck and prevent me from developing bed sores or poor circulation. The highlight of my week became my massage, which did wonders for my stiff muscles and provided me with an hour of company and conversation. A few weeks into bed rest and massage therapy, my masseuse informed me that she was pregnant. When I asked her if she could continue to come over, she, who was grossly obese and had to carry and set up a table and massage me, said sure, no problem. She planned to work until she gave birth. It seemed to me that everyone but me felt fully confident in the success of her pregnancy and immune to any problems.

The first few weeks of bed rest passed uneventfully. I read a lot, saw many movies, gabbed on the phone, picked up a bit of Spanish, and entertained visitors. Since she knew that I was on house arrest and I could no longer get away with screening calls, my mother-in-law called regularly to interrogate me and check to see if I was still pregnant. In fact, for weeks she would question whether I was "really" pregnant. "Are you sure the test was accurate?" she would ask. She even wondered if I could be partially pregnant. Despite reassurances that I had had many tests and seen pictures of the fetus, she wasn't entirely convinced. In contrast to the unpleasant harassment of my mother-in-law, one friend, to whom I feel forever grateful, visited me every weekday. She graciously dropped by, often with food or supplies, and provided delightful company. I credit her with helping me maintain some level of sanity throughout the entire confinement period. Other friends visited and brought lunch or movies. It wasn't really that unpleasant at times. The highlight of every week, besides the masseuse, was my doctor appointment. Once a week I saw either the perinatologist, the obstetrician, or had an ultrasound. Basically, I was monitored by someone every week. This meant that I could actually go outside and see the exciting sites of my neighborhood and different people. Although I had had enough of doctors and hospitals by this point, I still looked forward to visiting them because it was my small dose of freedom from bed rest.

I became strangely attentive to my surroundings when I was trapped alone in the house all of the time. I learned when our neighbors' gardeners arrived, who had children, when they went to and returned from school, who had dogs, and how often fire engines and police sirens went by. I also came to loathe one of my neighbors. From what I could determine, from spending many days of listening to them, my neighbor is a single father with two young boys. The father worked at the local university and appeared to have most of the summer off during which time he hung out at home, opened all of his windows, and blasted World Music throughout his house and into mine. He also hosted weekly all-day long parties in his backyard. From my eavesdropping, I concluded that after he and his children were abandoned by his wife, he gained primary custody of his kids, who more or less amused themselves and ran wild in their backyard and sometimes ours, a mere few feet away from my perch on the sofa situated next to a window that faces his house. Since I didn't know his name, I couldn't call him, and he couldn't hear me screaming "shut up" over his music. To me, he came to represent all that was wrong with the world and, specifically, he exemplified bad parenting. He was a semi-negligent parent, careless, rude, and self-righteous, who in my mind was hardly fit to have children. Although I undoubtedly projected a great deal of anger and frustration onto a semi-stranger, I do feel somewhat justified in demonizing him. It's been quite a while since I've been off bed rest and out of the house, and he's still an obnoxious neighbor.

Since I was confined to bed, I became what I swore I would never become—an internet junkie. I spent hours a day Googling everyone I had ever met. It was as if finding out information about people, even if inaccurate or outdated, was compensation for my limited human interaction while lounging in bed. It gave me the illusion that I was still in the loop socially. I also emailed tons of acquaintances and participated in instant messaging with good friends. Despite being bored and curious, I wasn't interested in talking computer to computer with people I hardly knew. Much to the dismay of my husband, I conducted quite a bit of online commerce. I bought maternity clothes and registered for baby gifts. A friend who had recently had a baby even came over to help me select the best and most useful baby items. I investigated baby furniture and bedding and became increasingly hopeful. Although I'm not superstitious, I kept telling myself that registering for baby supplies wouldn't jinx the pregnancy but instead, would ensure its success.

I also used my free time to research medical sites on bed rest and incompetent cervix. Most of what I read confirmed what I already knew, but it was helpful to reread statistics that gave me good odds and justified the decision I had made. I was disturbed, however, to read about all of the controversies surrounding the prescription of bed rest. It usually worked, but no one was really certain why it was helpful in some cases or even if bed rest was healthy, particularly for the mother, and ultimately beneficial. Having information gave me the illusion that I had some control over my pregnancy and its outcome. Like the doctors who ordered bed rest, I was doing something. I also glanced at chat rooms for pregnant women on bed rest but never participated and soon quit even visiting them. It was small comfort to me to know that there were lots of pregnant women confined to bed for one reason or another. It seemed as if obstetrics had returned to treatments of a previous age for lack of any proven, scientific remedies.

For the first week and a half of bed rest I felt fine and Dr. M. thought that everything looked normal after my post-cerclage appointment with her. Early the next morning after my medical exam I noticed that I was bleeding. I promptly called my obstetrician who told me to go to the hospital for an ultrasound. Bleeding, she said, was never a good sign, though it wasn't necessarily a bad sign. She would alert the perinatologist. As luck would have it, Roger was away for the day, so I called a friend who drove me to the hospital. Again, I walked the lengthy corridors to the ultrasound area, past the NICU. It seemed strange to me that no one, not one of my many doctors, suggested I use a wheelchair when attending appointments at the large hospital. Was it really good for me to be walking that much? I also hadn't figured out a route to the ultrasound section that didn't involve going down two steps. How would I do that in a wheelchair? Once again, I thought, the rules of bed rest are very nebulous. To make matters worse, there were no empty seats in the waiting area. Even though most of the people sitting in the room were not pregnant or infirm, no one offered his or her chair, so I had to sit on the floor. I had come to the conclusion that the hospital employed many fine doctors and nurses but needed to invest a bit in its waiting areas. The ultrasound indicated that everything was fine.

There was no evidence of bleeding, the baby's heart rate was good, and my cervix looked long and closed. So I returned home mystified but somewhat comforted.

Later that day the perinatologist called and wanted to see me immediately. A friend had stopped by while I was on the phone with the doctor, so I corralled her into taking me back to the hospital. For the second time that day I walked down another long corridor to Dr. D.'s office. He examined me and determined that my cervix was indeed still closed but that Dr. M. had probably rattled the stitches when she had examined me the previous day, which had caused the bleeding. He sent me home to rest some more and called Dr. M. to chastise her. This time I did not have a cavalier attitude or try to rationalize why I was bleeding. I had taken action immediately and everything turned out well. Probably I was just lucky this time.

After a few uneventful weeks on bed rest, I got to return for the umpteenth time for another ultrasound—a level two ultrasound to determine if the baby was developing normally. For the second time, we found out that our daughter's organs were perfectly formed; she appeared to be healthy and growing beautifully. My cervix still appeared to be long and closed. I reminded myself that I just had to get through at least twelve or thirteen more weeks and the baby was likely to be okay. I was fairly confident that I could manage it.

Many women experience various digestive problems when pregnant like gas, bloating, and constipation. I had during my first pregnancy, but this round it was infinitely worse. I suspect that eating while horizontal and rarely walking exacerbated my condition. Shortly after the level-two ultrasound, I began to have terrible pain in my abdomen. It felt like a gastro-intestinal problem, but I couldn't be certain. At the advice of my obstetrician, I was already taking Metamucil and Colace and showing no improvement. At times, the pain was excruciating. So once again, off I went to the hospital. I was admitted to labor and delivery and after being examined by various doctors and residents, was sent to have another ultrasound. The doctors looked for ruptured ovaries and tumors and burst appendix. Nothing! Everything looked normal. I ended up spending two nights in the hospital—one in a labor and delivery room and one in the maternity ward. I was still in some pain, but no one could figure out what was wrong. So I was discharged and told to continue taking Metamucil and Colace. The pain never really went away completely, but I muddled through and every doctor insisted that everything appeared to be just great.

At about the twenty-first week of pregnancy all of my doctors, and I had many, went on vacation. Dr. D. was in South Africa for a few weeks and Dr. M. and her sister, who was in practice with her and usually covered for her when she was away, were going to Spain for a family gathering. While everyone was gone I was monitored by the Fellow in perinatology, Dr. L., as well as the usual ultrasound doctors and technicians. Despite liking the Fellow and trusting that she was competent, I was not thrilled that my regular doctors would be out of the country as I was approaching my twenty-fourth week of pregnancy. I had gone into labor once before around this time and I was becoming increasingly nervous as that week loomed. I wanted to believe that if I could get past that marker, everything would be alright.

At about 5:00 PM, two days shy of my twenty-third week of pregnancy, my water broke when I was using the bathroom. "Here we go again," I thought, calm, cool, and still rational. As I emerged from the bathroom, I told Roger in a flat, what-else-is-new voice, "It's all over. My water just broke. We need to go to the hospital." I called Labor and Delivery to let them know we were on our way and drove off to see the maternity staff, who were now beginning to seem like old friends. After checking in, I was again placed in a labor and delivery room where I was hooked up to various monitors and examined. The baby still had a heartbeat, but it was not as strong as it should be. Her umbilical cord had evidently detached and emerged when my water broke, which meant that the baby would probably die soon since she had no lifeline. Although my cervix was dilated, it wasn't sufficiently dilated for me to give birth, and I was only just starting to have contractions. So all there was to do was wait. The other problem was that none of my doctors was available. The staff placed calls to various other doctors who were supposed to be covering for them but failed to reach anyone. The residents didn't want to deal with me because I was a high-risk case and because I informed them that my obstetrician had told me in no uncertain terms that I had to have a C-section. Apparently, there was some controversy among the doctors on call about this. Also, that evening the maternity ward was particularly busy. There were many women about to give birth to live, healthy babies. Basically, I just lay on the bed and was monitored for hours while various doctors and nurses dropped in to check on my progress.

When my cervix had dilated further and the contractions were getting stronger and more frequent I was wheeled into another room and hooked up to more monitors. The anesthesiologist and a resident came by to offer me an epidural, which I gladly accepted. After poking around my spine for a while, I was finally numbed effectively and again left to recline for a while longer. An epidural dulls the pain of contractions and makes it bearable but certainly doesn't obliterate it. At last, I was sufficiently dilated and so another Fellow in perinatology, who looked like she'd been on call for days, came in to deliver the baby. She insisted that there was no need for a C-section since the baby was so small my uterus wouldn't tear, and there was no chance of her surviving any kind of delivery. So I pushed her out relatively easily. The doctor wanted to know if Roger and I wanted to see the baby before she was taken away. We both promptly responded, "No." Neither of us had any desire to see a dead baby. Why didn't anyone get it that it was not helpful to hold a dying baby or see a stillborn? Why would I want to get attached to or have to keep picturing dead infants? The doctor informed us about our options for what to do with the baby's body. We opted for cremation this time. We were not having a funeral, memorial service, or burial, and we were not naming her. Since she was stillborn, there was no need for a death certificate and therefore no birth certificate.

I was later wheeled into a private room in the maternity ward as I had been after giving birth to Emily. The hospital certainly did its best to avoid putting women who had lost babies in rooms with women and their newborns. Roger told me that there was a black strip on the doorpost of my room as a warning sign to doctors and nurses that our baby had died. It felt to me like the mark of Cain. In fact, the next morning when one of the doctors, whom I had met a number of times and who had done one of my ultrasounds and who was a perinatologist, was making his rounds, paused by my door and walked away. I guess he felt that he had nothing to check on. I had no baby and had had a relatively easy delivery, medically speaking, and I was being discharged later that day. The black sign warned people to keep away from me. Perhaps the black mark and I represented his and his colleagues' failures to bring my pregnancy to term and deliver a live baby. I definitely felt like the hospital staff was avoiding me. Maybe no one could bear the awful task of saying, "I'm sorry for your loss" and being unable to remedy the situation.

Early that morning when Roger went to the hospital cafeteria to get himself some coffee, he ran into the high-risk pregnancy Fellow, Dr. L., who was covering for my perinatologist. She had never been called the night before and had no idea that I'd gone into pre-term labor and given birth. He described her reaction as shocked and horrified. After I'd been discharged that afternoon she called me at home to talk about what happened and let me know that she had stopped by to see me, but I'd already been discharged. She urged me to call Dr. D. when he returned from vacation to discuss what had happened and to see if he had any insights about it. Also, she said that I could ask him about other options if I wanted to try to have another child. What would he do next, sew up my entire uterus and hang me upside down for six months? That was not the day to talk to me about being pregnant again. I felt totally deflated and had no faith in any doctor's powers. I certainly was not about to go on bed rest again, pointlessly, and experience yet more heartache.

## Chapter 4

Because, to some degree, I'd been through this before and knew it was a possibility, losing our second baby was less shocking than losing the first. The combination of bed rest, followed by preterm labor, a vaginal delivery, a stillborn baby, and a mere nineteen-hour hospital stay made for a surreal experience. After being discharged from the hospital Roger and I remembered that our housekeepers would be cleaning our home that day. We weren't in the mood to explain what happened and knew that they were likely to get very emotional and start crying when they heard our news, especially since they too had gone through similar experiences many years ago. So to kill time and avoid our house and social interaction, but still get away from the hospital, we went out to lunch at a local diner. It was exceptionally weird dining in public after having been confined in the house for months and after just losing a baby. I imagine that we appeared relatively normal. Perhaps we seemed a bit down, and I was moving slowly and looked a bit disheveled in my maternity clothes, but nothing really out of the ordinary. So there we sat, as if everything were fine, near other people on their lunch breaks.

Despite having spent over eleven weeks in bed, I recovered physically much more quickly this round since I did not have another C-section. Although I lacked my usual energy and muscle tone, I was not in pain every time I turned or got up from a chair, and was more than eager to get out of the house for a stroll. My psychological recovery was easier this time as well. Really knowing what to expect and not expect when you're expecting prevented the shock and denial I underwent after my first loss. This time I was terribly disappointed, resigned, and frustrated. I was particularly angry that medicine had failed me once again. I was also certain that I would never be pregnant again. I was unwilling to undergo any more elective surgical procedures and follow dubious medical advice knowing that it was unlikely to enable me to have a baby. When I agreed to have a cerclage and stay on bed rest it was with the understanding that I was likely to carry to at least thirty-two weeks. My odds were good. Now it was very clear that my cervix was highly incompetent—so much so that it busted open the stitches and began dilating. My odds of carrying a baby to term were now very poor.

Shortly after I returned home from the hospital I left a message with my obstetrician about what had happened. She called me as soon as she returned and wanted to see me. Dr. M. was very upset about my going into pre-term labor again and that no one had called Dr. L., the Fellow and

Dr. D.'s substitute, when I was in labor. She was outraged that a stranger delivered my baby despite the fact that I knew many of the obstetricians and perinatologists affiliated with the hospital. She too had no answers or solutions as to why the cerclage and bed rest didn't work, and she recommended that I call Dr. D. and discuss the matter with him. Dr. M. also suggested that I look into using a gestational surrogate should I decide to try to have a baby again. Basically, I was fertile and capable of producing healthy babies but unable to carry them, so a surrogate might be the perfect solution to my problem. Dr. M. gave me the contact information of a patient of hers who had used a gestational carrier if I wanted some information about surrogacy, and referrals to a number of fertility doctors and clinics. At that point I still wanted an explanation about what had gone wrong before I was ready to leap into action and come up with a new plan.

Inspired by Dr. M. and determined to get some answers, I called Dr. D.'s office and explained my situation and that Dr. L. had urged me to call. I talked Dr. D.'s nurse at length who agreed that I should speak with Dr. D.; she promised me to give him my message. He did not return my call. I called two more times and was assured that he would call me back or the nurse would call me to set up a time to speak with him. I never heard from them again. When I was pregnant, Dr. D. was attentive and available; however, now that he was clearly unable to help me and had failed in his mission to maintain my pregnancy, he wanted nothing to do with me. I had no interest in blaming him for this pregnancy failure. I simply wanted his insights as to what went wrong and why. I wanted to know if I had any other options. Dr. D. was undoubtedly a very busy man, but he still owed me the courtesy of returning my phone calls and finishing the job that, as far as I was concerned, he had not completed.

I was absolutely furious. I wanted a logical, scientific explanation for why my cervix dilated despite the cerclage and why I even had an incompetent cervix. What triggered my cervix to dilate? It seemed unlikely to me that it was the weight of the baby. I was never that big, and I was on bed rest during the second pregnancy; there wasn't that much weight pressing down on my cervix. Maybe my cervix was just extraordinarily incompetent. Even that seemed odd since I had never had any procedures or trauma, like cancer or an abortion that might weaken my cervix. It appeared to me that something chemical was triggering my going into labor. When I suggested this, doctors looked at me as if I were a fool or simply shrugged their shoulders or dismissed me. Also women who appeared to be in much worse shape than I was—women who had no cervixes or serious other complications or illnesses in addition to cervical incompetence, managed to carry to term with medical intervention and bed rest—so why couldn't I? To this day, I have yet to receive a satisfactory explanation.

The intensive monitoring of my second pregnancy also seemed pointless and provided no answers or remedies. I had ultrasounds just about every week, sometimes a few times a week, from about the eighth week to the end of my second pregnancy. The ultrasounds provided me and the doctors with many interesting pictures of the developing baby but were in no way predictive of the course of my pregnancy. They simply showed what was going at the time of the ultrasound. As a matter of fact, they weren't even that accurate. Each time I went in for an ultrasound, my cervix was measured. It was always deemed to be sufficiently long and closed. Sometimes it even seemed to have grown longer, which was clearly ridiculous. Apparently, depending on the angle of the picture, the cervix can appear to be longer or shorter. So the measurements were not really precise at all. Perhaps they could simply determine whether my cervix looked okay and closed versus dangerously short and opened. Also, what would they do if it were dilating? I had been told the first time that I went into early labor that once I started dilating, nothing could be done to stop the dilation. Other than depicting what was happening at a particular moment, what use was ultrasound in terms of preventing my going into pre-term labor? In my second pregnancy, I had my last ultrasound when I was over twenty-two weeks along and everything looked fine. A few days later, I went into labor. Obviously, my cervix dilated quickly and spontaneously. If the ultrasound wasn't scheduled for the day that my cervix happened to open, well, then, I was out of luck. Besides, what could be done at that point anyway?

One evening, around the time of my calling assault on Dr. D., Roger and I took a stroll around our neighborhood. As we were walking, we noticed a short, rotund fellow wearing a fluorescent reflective vest coming towards us, and laughed at the sight. As he approached us we realized that it was none other than Dr. D. who nodded at us with an "I've-seen-you somewhere-before" look and continued on his way. I was fuming and stunned. Did he think we were one of his neighbors? How could he not know that I was his patient and had been trying to reach him for days? Did he only recognize me by my uterus?

About a week later, Labor Day weekend, Roger and I decided to escape for a few days to a nearby hotel and resort and do our best to forget about our travails. The weather was lovely, and we had a relaxing time hiking, eating, and lounging. On the last morning of our stay, we had brunch in the dining room, and while surveying the treats on the buffet table, I noticed Dr. D. from the corner of my eye. I purposely lurked by the table, hoping to catch his attention, but he walked by either avoiding me or simply not noticing me. Later that day on a walk, Roger and I bumped into Dr. D. again, who merely smiled at us in recognition and kept walking. I wonder if he thought we were stalking him or really had no idea who we were or that we were disappointed and frustrated former patients of his. Over the years we've run into Dr. D. numerous times, at the movies, in restaurants, and on walks. We were even seated right next to him at a Thai restaurant in our neighborhood. He showed no evidence of recognizing us in the least. I guess after a while all of his former patients have blurred together. He fixes or fails to fix a problem and moves on. I hadn't and was still miffed at him for neglecting to return my calls.

After the second loss I found it even more difficult to enjoy social interaction and go about my daily routines. No place was safe; almost everything and everywhere were saturated with pregnancy-related associations. Many women at my gym had already given birth to one or two children in the time that I had lost two. It seemed that almost everyone I knew was pregnant or had babies. Since I had taken the year off, I had few distractions and too much time to stew. In part, as a diversion, I enrolled in an adult education Spanish class at the local university. I had hoped and assumed that an introductory Spanish course would be a maternity-discussion-free zone and that I could focus on verb conjugations and information about Spanish-speaking countries instead of pregnancy losses. However, no sooner than the second day of class, everyone had to introduce him or herself, including information about one's career and family. We had just learned the word "jubilado" meaning retired, which applied to an eighty-year old member of the class. Because I didn't know how to say "I'm on a failed maternity leave," I too became "jubilada," although I was by no means jubilant about it. We also learned the words for various family members and were asked if we had children. When I studied French in high school no one assumed that I had children, and so it didn't occur to me that this would be a topic for discussion in a basic language class. So I had to confess that I had no children and no job. There was no safety zone. Also, when I met people at parties or work-related events for Roger, they would inevitably ask what I did and when I said that I was taking the year off, would follow with, "Do you have children?" It is assumed that if you are an educated female professional who is not working, you must be taking time off to raise children. I always answered "no" and probably winced and changed the subject quickly. I've been asked that question hundreds of times.

And then of course, again, I felt envious of and mystified by all of my friends and acquaintances who had problem-free pregnancies and believed that nothing could possibly go wrong. After my second pregnancy fiasco I gave all of my maternity clothes, which I could not bear to look at, to a friend from work, who was due around the same time I would have been. At twenty-five weeks pregnant, she insisted on hauling the large bags of clothes to her car by herself, confident in her body's powers. How could she be certain that doing heavy lifting wouldn't cause a problem? How could she, who had never been pregnant before, be so sure that she would carry to forty weeks? And yet she did, and like so many other women, wasn't particularly worried that anything would go wrong. When I was first pregnant, I wasn't overly nervous and pretty much assumed the best. But now, despite plenty of evidence to the contrary, I can't understand how or believe that anyone carries to term and delivers a healthy baby.

Since it was becoming clear that I wasn't getting any satisfactory explanations about my pregnancy losses any time soon, I did some research on my own and got busy with a new plan. It turns out that there is a more radical form of cerclage, a transabdominal cerclage, that is permanent, more complicated, involves a laparotomy, and is not that frequently performed, and best of all, is not necessarily efficacious; no doubt, it includes bed rest too. I was sure that I would not undergo such an ordeal. It seemed like voluntary mutilation and martyrdom to me and there was no guarantee that it would work anyway. Basically, I had to acknowledge that I would never be pregnant again and possibly never have my own biological child. Since pregnancy itself was mostly a negative experience for me, I was relieved not to enter into that miserable, and to me, pointless, state yet again. However, the idea of not having a child with Roger's and my genes was harder to accept, particularly since we had come so close. Perhaps if I had been infertile and had never conceived and carried two babies, I would have been more amenable to adoption or even remaining childless. But I had lost something, and I felt that I had something to fix. Our two remaining options seemed to be gestational surrogacy or adoption.

Acting quickly made me feel better. It was certainly preferable to passively moping or fuming at home. My new job became researching surrogacy and adoption. I read books and articles, talked to doctors, lawyers, friends, and friends of friends. Each side had its pros and cons. I looked into both domestic and foreign adoption. Domestic adoption was the first option we ruled out. The trend towards open adoption made me very uncomfortable, as did having anything to do with the birth mother even after the child turned eighteen. I was also haunted by the idea that the birth mother could change her mind even after the baby was born. I was also repelled by the many websites of various adoption lawyers in which desperate couples advertised themselves to prospective birth mothers. There was no way that I would compete on line and so overtly with other couples for a child by telling my sob story and describing my house and job and including a cute photo of Roger and me. I was also turned off after talking to a prominent adoption lawyer in northern California who made it clear that I would do all of the work—advertising, interviewing, pretty much everything but the contract, for which she would be paid large sums of money. It seemed that domestic adoption, particularly through private lawyers, lacks privacy and a sense of dignity and discretion.

I liked the anonymity of foreign adoption but was concerned about the care of the babies and their health. In the end, I crossed Russia and Ukraine off my list after reading horror stories about babies with fetal alcohol syndrome neglected in terrible orphanages and the egregious red tape of those governments. I also heard mixed reports about adopting from South and Central America, so I, like so many other women of my class, homed in on adopting a little girl from China. While I had some concerns about adoption in general and from China in particular, I was willing to pursue it further. Roger, however, was less enthusiastic. He saw adoption as a last resort. Perhaps because he is an only child whose father is no longer alive he felt a greater need than I to carry on his line. He had concerns about a child who looked nothing like us and whose family background and medical history were unknown. Engineer and techie that he is, Roger contended that we had the materials with which to create a child; we just needed a carrier. Consequently, he preferred to have a child by means whose variables he could control than through adoption, over which he could have no input. There are times that I wish we had explored adoption more thoroughly. But for us, at that time, adoption didn't feel like the best choice, so we focused our energies on surrogacy.

Despite or because it's less popular, surrogacy was easier to research and involved fewer choices. On the surface, it sounded like the perfect solution for us. We could provide the raw materials, an egg and sperm, and the surrogate would provide a functioning uterus that could hold the baby for nine months. In gestational surrogacy the carrier serves as a host uterus for the egg and sperm of a couple or of donors and involves in vitro fertilization. In traditional surrogacy, the carrier is artificially inseminated with the father's sperm. It seemed nuts to me that I, an English Ph.D., wanna-be Luddite, who views a computer as a necessary evil, uses a cell phone only for emergencies, and has no interest in owning a Blackberry or Ipod and other high-tech gadgets, would be having a high-tech baby.

Like many people of my generation, the first thing I thought of when I heard the term surrogacy was the Baby M. case of the 1980's. My hazy recollections of the news reports of the case involved a crazy surrogate who refused to give up the child to the intended mother. I had no idea if I was remembering the case accurately, but I was certainly worried about dealing with a surrogate who would get attached to my baby after having carried it for nine months and refuse to give it to us. It turns out that the Baby M. case was a traditional surrogacy in which Mary Beth Whitehead, the surrogate, was the biological mother of the child. Also, the intended mother's name did not appear in the contract. Since we weren't going to be using traditional surrogacy and hoped to have a good lawyer, clear, well-written contracts, and an emotionally stable gestational surrogate, my concerns were somewhat alleviated. Also, after talking to a lawyer and some surrogacy agencies, I learned that surrogacy laws, especially in California, are much more straightforward and in some ways, easier, than adoption laws. There were no recent cases in which the surrogate wanted to keep the baby.

The most complicated part of surrogacy was the medical procedures. I would have to undergo the first part of IVF, meaning weeks of hormone shots and a surgery to retrieve my eggs, but instead of transferring the embryos to my uterus, they'd be placed in that of another woman who would carry them for the duration of the pregnancy. So much for my vow to have nothing to do with IVF. The surrogate would also be subjected to weeks of hormone injections to prepare her body for pregnancy. I hadn't yet committed to using a gestational carrier but was actively researching and pursuing it. I was determined to have a baby one way or another, and this seemed like the most promising and appropriate approach for us.

## Chapter 5

*O*ur first step in the quest for a surrogate was a consultation with a fertility doctor in San Francisco, who had experience working with gestational surrogates. Dr. M. had referred us to him in the hope that he could explain the process of in vitro fertilization with a gestational surrogate, to determine whether or not we were good candidates for such an undertaking, and to refer us to a surrogacy agency and a lawyer who specialized in this field. The fertility center was quite the place, situated in a modern building complex with breathtaking views of the Bay and a smartly decorated office with sleek furniture and modern art. I couldn't help but wonder if the consultation fee wouldn't have been lower had we not been paying for the center's expensive décor. It seemed to me that there had to be a happy medium between this overly posh waiting area that looked like the lobby of a slick hotel and the sparsely furnished, mildewed waiting rooms at the hospital. The fertility doctor, Dr. C. was charming and helpful. After reviewing my medical records and discussing our situation, he concluded that we'd be fine candidates for working with a surrogate. He then recommended an agency in another part of the Bay Area, and we were on our way.

As soon as we got home, I called the agency to set up a consultation. The head of the agency, to whom I was immediately connected, was exceedingly enthusiastic, encouraging, and informative. Her strong sales pitch and seeming desperation for clients brought out the skeptic in me, but I decided to stick with the appointment. I had little to lose and might be pleasantly surprised. The next day we received an information packet in the mail from the agency. Her promptness was impressive but a bit much. I wondered if she dropped off the packet on our doorstep herself. The informational literature was decorated with the logo of the agency—intertwining hearts--- and included touching stories of formerly childless couples who were now blessed with babies who had been carried by surrogates. Mrs. B., the founder and director and, from what I could determine, sole employee of the agency, had quite a bit of experience in the field and was anything but a disinterested bureaucrat. In this situation my concern was no longer the prospect of dealing with an aloof, insensitive doctor but with a mother hen who would micromanage every facet of the surrogacy process, treat me like a child, and drive me nuts. My skepticism was growing by the minute, but I was determined at least to go through with the consultation.

The agency was located in a small, bland office in non-descript office park in a suburb of San Francisco. When we arrived for our meeting we were greeted warmly by an administrative assistant, whom I believe was the only other employee of the agency. We were immediately ushered into a small conference room and offered beverages and snacks, and given lots of paperwork to read and fill out. Mrs. B. would see us shortly. Mrs. B. was much as I had imagined her—mid fifties but looked older, haircut and clothing of the nineteen-eighties, and a doting manner. We chatted with her for a while and explained our situation in detail. She then went over the reams of paper and explained the legal, medical, and financial aspects of surrogacy. The agency had a number of available and screened surrogates from whom we could choose. After being selected, our potential surrogate would be sent information about us and a video in which we would introduce ourselves and tell our story. Roger and I looked at each other at the mention of the video. Neither one of us was too keen about being filmed, but we nodded and smiled, hoping to learn more.

Then Mrs. B. took out a binder that included surrogate profiles and invited us to look through it. She would leave the room for a while and let us peruse the files of her available surrogates. The profiles include photos and personal and medical information. I was taken aback that she would entrust us with such information. It felt like we were violating the privacy of these women; we hadn't even signed on with the agency and she was already sharing information about people's families, their religious views, and medical histories. I was not overly impressed with the collection of surrogates or the screening process. One of them admitted to being a smoker, but wrote that she would quit if she got pregnant. Another had had three abortions before she was married and now asserted that every life was sacred and that under no circumstances would she terminate a pregnancy. Clearly she wanted to be a surrogate for all the wrong reasons, namely, to make up for the pregnancies she aborted and to expiate her guilt. Mrs. B. definitely needed a better screening process and perhaps even to employ a psychologist to help determine the motives and psychological stability of the surrogates as well as the intended parents.

After our exhaustive and exhausting search through the binder, Mrs. B. returned to check on us and see if we'd found anyone we liked. We hesitatingly named one woman who was a single mother and full-time student, but we were concerned that she had no support system and a great many responsibilities. Mrs. B. assured us not to worry. She would take care of everything. I felt like I was adopting a new mother rather than a surrogate. Then, once again, Mrs. B. brought up the dreaded video. She brightly suggested that we film it immediately. Roger and I should jot down some notes, and I could touch up my lipstick and action! At that point her enthusiasm and eagerness to close the deal were getting on our nerves. As a united front Roger and I explained that we wanted time to think about whether to proceed with surrogacy and would call her when we were ready to shoot a video. She insisted that there was no time like the present and continued her sales pitch, but Roger and I stood firm. We barely escaped unshot and unsigned. Needless to say, we left with a "we'll be in touch" and little intention of returning. Oddly enough, though we were unlikely to use this agency, we weren't completely discouraged. We'd learned a great deal of information about the process and still had other resources and options. We were quite relieved to escape Mrs. B.'s clutches.

Next, I called Dr. M.'s patient who had used a surrogate and recently had a baby. She was very helpful and informative. She strongly recommended that I contact the surrogacy agency that she used, which was based in Los Angeles. She had nothing but praise for the agency and its large staff and many resources. The agency, which has been around since the early days of surrogacy, helps provide legal counsel, locate and arrange fertility and other medical treatments, employs full-time psychologists and social workers, and is well managed and effective. This certainly sounded like an improvement over Mrs. B.'s one-woman operation. While talking with her, I could hear her newborn cooing in the background. Here was living proof that surrogacy could really work. This woman was the only person I'd ever spoken to who used a surrogate, and she sounded sane and intelligent. I was encouraged. For a moment I didn't feel like I was participating in some controversial science experiment. Having a baby with a surrogate was plausible and reasonable.

The one thing that made me uncomfortable in my conversation with this woman was her frequent declarations about her infertility and her assumptions about mine. Her language was loaded with infertility jargon that made her sound as if she attended weekly support groups that inspired her to make daily affirmations about her fertility status. She evidently wasn't completely infertile since she'd used her own eggs to have her baby. Perhaps the term "infertility" was now being loosely applied to anyone who has had any problems of any kind conceiving, carrying, or delivering a baby. I didn't consider myself infertile and neither did any of my doctors. I wonder if confessing to infertility makes women believe that they can remedy any maternity problems. I came close to interrupting and correcting her but thought better of it. She had been helpful, and it wasn't for me to disrupt her infertility mantra if it made her feel better. But it did make me wonder what I was getting into.

I immediately investigated the Los Angeles-based surrogacy agency on line. Their website is thorough and useful, and the agency has been operating since the dawn of surrogacy. So, once again, I mustered up some more courage and called the agency for information and to set up a consultation. I was connected to the director of the agency who spent a great deal of time on the phone with me discussing my options, telling me about surrogacy, the agency, and answering any questions I had. Her manner was friendly yet professional, which I liked. She said that she'd send me an information packet and told me that the agency requires clients to come to their office in LA for a day-long series of meetings and information sessions with various members of the staff, including a lawyer and psychologist. Despite the inconvenience of flying down to LA, I was impressed that this agency screened its clients and wanted them to be well informed about what they were undertaking. They were also good at marketing themselves; nonetheless, after receiving the information pack, I set up an appointment with them, sent off the necessary paperwork, medical records, and information about ourselves, and planned a little trip to Los Angeles.

When we arrived for our induction at the LA agency, we were greeted by a receptionist, who ushered us into a conference room, offered us coffee, and gave Roger and me our schedules for the day and an information packet. Once again, we had a great deal of paperwork to fill out and read. Throughout the day we were to meet with various members of the staff who would discuss their particular roles and areas of expertise in the surrogacy process. We first met with a warm, gracious woman whose job was to introduce new clients to the world of surrogacy. She, herself had two children through a gestational surrogate many years ago. This woman did a wonderful job of alleviating many of our anxieties about surrogacy. She explained the process by which couples were matched with a surrogate. Surrogates are given extensive psychological and medical screening. They, along with their spouses or partners, are interviewed by staff psychologists. All surrogates have to have at least one child of their own and a history of problem-free pregnancies. Basically, the agency wanted to insure that the surrogates were stable, had the support of their partners, were healthy, and not interested in keeping another couple's baby. Already, many of my anxieties were alleviated. The surrogate was unlikely to want to keep our baby and she wouldn't be smoking and drinking her way through the pregnancy.

Couples were matched with surrogates based on certain shared values, sometimes geographical considerations, and practical pregnancy-related and medical concerns. For instance, in our case, we would be paired with a surrogate from California, who would agree to terminate a pregnancy if medically necessary, and would undergo prenatal genetic testing. The agency would match a few couples with a particular surrogate who would then be given those couples' files and get to choose which one she wants to work with. Once the surrogate makes her selection, the couple is notified and sent information about the surrogate. When all parties express interest, the agency arranges a meeting which is mediated initially by one of the agency psychologists or counselors. If everyone likes each other and feels comfortable with the match, contracts and medical appointments are arranged, and the process gets underway.

We continued to talk with the same woman, who answered our questions and understood our concerns about surrogacy. She made one particular comment, which I still think about. She said that while we undergo this process, friends, family, and even brief acquaintances will ask us why we don't just adopt and why we bother to go through the trouble and expense of using a surrogate. She advised that we hold firm and just ask them if they have children of their own, and if so, why they didn't adopt instead. She emphasized that no one else, especially someone who had children easily, is in a position to pass judgment. Since then, I've been questioned and challenged many times about my decision to use a surrogate and always by someone who has a bunch of kids or by an idealistic, single friend with no children, who believes that adoption is the most ethical option. I have been grateful for the comeback.

We then met with a financial advisor, a medical coordinator, and a former surrogate. The financial advisor explained the numerous costs and payment schedules. In addition to the agency, legal, medical, and counseling fees, we would put money into a trust for the surrogate from which she'd be compensated and reimbursed throughout her pregnancy and the entire surrogacy process. Once we were matched with a surrogate, we would choose a fertility clinic that was convenient for the surrogate and us and go on from there. I was tremendously relieved to meet the former surrogate. She seemed perfectly sane, intelligent, and pleasant. Although I'm sure that she'd been asked this a million times before, I couldn't help questioning her about why she wanted to be a surrogate or for that matter why would anyone want to carry a baby for a perfect stranger. I couldn't even carry my own babies and had unpleasant pregnancy experiences, so from my perspective, no reasonable person would volunteer to do this for someone else. The surrogate explained that she loved being pregnant, never had any problems, and felt that it was something she could do well and a gift that she could give others. She also said that she had loved ones who had fertility problems or couldn't have children and felt a strong need to help couples who couldn't have children on their own. Also, it was a way for some women to earn some money while raising their own families. Even though I could in no way identify with what this woman said and her self-sacrifice, I respected her beliefs and was grateful that she and other women like her existed.

After a nice lunch break, we met with the head psychologist of the agency. She explained the screening process in more detail and told us about the counselor's role in the whole surrogacy process. Each couple and surrogate would be assigned a counselor who would serve as an advisor, intermediary, sounding board, and someone to help ease the way through the whole ordeal. The counselors were also responsible for screening couples and surrogates and for matching them. We were told that it would take approximately three to six months to be paired with a surrogate. We were also told that we would be a particularly easy case since we were relatively young, had especially heartbreaking experiences, were fertile, and lived in California. Apparently, many surrogates would want to work with us since they were likely to get pregnant relatively easily given that we had no history of fertility problems and were under forty. We lived in a surrogacy-friendly state, and our pathetic story would appeal to many a hopeful and idealistic surrogate. I was impressed by the strong support system that the agency provided both to the couples and the surrogates. I was also encouraged by the psychologist's words; apparently we were the ideal candidates to work with a surrogate. I do wonder if she told that to most of her potential clients.

We then met with an attorney who specializes in surrogacy law. He assured us that we had little to be concerned about vis a vis surrogacy in California. He had written hundreds of surrogacy contracts, and none had been challenged. He went over the contracts in detail and allayed my fears about Baby M. The last person we met with was the founder and head of the agency, who mostly seemed to want to entertain us and check us out. He had a fine sense of humor, was very engaging, and did a great job closing the deal. Before we left for the day, we got a chance to ask any remaining questions of the woman who first introduced us to the agency. She also explained that once we had retained the agency we would need to write a profile of ourselves in the form of a letter to a potential surrogate. We should tell her a little about ourselves and our experiences and include a few photos. This was a vast improvement over being filmed. Roger and I are no actors, but we could easily write a little story about ourselves. This approach made us far more comfortable. By the end of our day-long orientation and interview, we were sold. After twenty-plus years in the surrogacy business, they seemed to have figured out what works and what doesn't. The agency was well run and appeared to know how to make the surrogacy process run smoothly and humanely for everyone involved. I was also pleased that they would provide a strong support system for Roger, me, and the surrogate and her family. For the first time in a long while, we felt encouraged and hopeful that we could have a child some time in the near future.

Shortly after we returned home, we filled out tons of paperwork, sent in retainers, took care of all of our medical screening and tests, composed our profile, and began our wait to be matched with a surrogate. Since we were such good candidates, we assumed that we would hear from the agency sooner rather than later. However, after hearing nothing from the agency for a few months, I panicked. Against my better judgment, I called the adoption lawyer I had spoken to earlier and disliked, in order to get information about scheduling a home visit by a social worker and beginning the adoption process. I wanted to cover my bases and at least get started on Plan B should I need it. Instead of answering my questions, the attorney interrogated me about surrogacy, asserted that the agency I was working with obviously wasn't doing a very good job, and that she, who handled surrogacy as well as adoption, could find me a surrogate immediately. Given that she does not find surrogates for her clients and made them do all the work, it seemed to me that under her guidance, I would search for and locate the surrogate myself and she would merely draft the contracts. She then urged me to set up a time to meet with her for a consultation, which was when I told her that I'd have to talk to my husband about it and hung up. I was outraged at her audacity to try to manipulate me and prey on my anxieties about surrogacy, adoption, and the LA agency by plugging her own services. Needless to say, we did not contact her again.

It had been six months, and we still hadn't heard a word from the surrogacy agency. So I called and was told by the woman whom we first met with that two of the surrogates that they had planned to match us with ended up having medical problems. Also, they were trying to find us a carrier who lived in northern California. I let her know that we didn't care if she lived near us, just preferably anywhere in the state of California. The agency representative continued that we were likely to be paired up shortly with someone who was currently undergoing medical and psychological screening. When I asked her why we weren't given updates or hadn't heard anything from the agency for so long, she explained that it wasn't their policy to update couples because it often created false hope and disappointment. They preferred to wait until they had a match, everyone was screened, and profiles had been sent. Her explanation was reasonable, but given that we had signed various retainers and sent thousands of dollars to the agency, they could, at the very least, have let us know that they were working on our case and hadn't forgotten us. Perhaps they could have sent a nice holiday card.

After eight months we finally received a call from the counselor assigned to us by the agency to let us know that we had been matched with a surrogate. While I was relieved to have a potential surrogate, I was annoyed that we had been kept waiting in the dark two months longer than the maximum amount of time we were told we would have to wait and five months longer than we were expecting and hoping to wait, especially since we had been informed that we were such an easy and appealing couple. Besides, I was approaching forty; my fertility clock was ticking, and I didn't have time to waste. The counselor, Susan, described the surrogate to us a bit and said that the surrogate was excited about us and hoped to work with us. Susan would forward the potential surrogate's profile, and if we were interested in her, we could set up a time to meet. There was one hitch: the surrogate lived in southern California and had four young children. If we wanted to work with her, we would have to use a fertility clinic within commuting distance of her home and have all procedures done in southern California. We could live with that arrangement. Our biggest concern was that we would like and trust the woman who might carry our baby.

Shortly after our conversation with the counselor, we received the surrogate's profile in the mail. Her profile included photos of her and her family, a letter in which she described herself, and medical information. The gestational surrogate, Donna, and her husband, Steve, live in southern California and have four young children, the youngest, twin boys. Steve is a plumber and Donna was a part-time escrow officer. In her enthusiastic and friendly letter she explained that she had wanted to be a surrogate for a long time, and now that she was done having children of her own she hoped to help another couple have a family. In describing her pregnancies, Donna repeatedly used the word "blessed," and added that "everything happens for a reason," when she referred to her third, and unplanned pregnancy with twins; these were red flags for me. I immediately assumed that she was overly religious and that I'd offend her with my cynicism and lack of belief in divine intervention. Roger, on the other hand, wasn't at all alarmed. In fact, he was relieved that she seemed stable and felt that she was just using some common expressions. It is possible that I was looking for ways in which Donna and I would be incompatible. No doubt I was ambivalent about using a surrogate and nervous about being able to trust her. I had to accept this complicated relationship with someone to whom I was both deeply grateful for being willing to carry our baby and also resentful of for taking my place.

My other concern about Donna's ability to be a good surrogate was that she had had two C-sections and delivered her twins at thirty-four weeks. Since my biggest fear was premature labor, the last thing I wanted to worry about in a surrogate was that she would deliver even a few weeks early. It turns out that Donna was induced because one twin was much smaller than the other. I called Dr. M. to ask about the multiple C-sections, scarring, and early delivery, and she reassured me that none of this was cause for concern or would affect Donna's ability to be a successful gestational surrogate. My other hesitation about Donna, which I was embarrassed to bring up to too many people other than Roger, was that she was quite overweight. I wanted to believe that she just hadn't taken off the extra weight she had gained from carrying twins only the previous year. But it did concern me that it put her at higher risk for carrying a pregnancy to term. Before agreeing to meet Donna and Steve, I basically had to take a leap of faith that she was stable, reasonable, tolerant, and had sound motives for undertaking surrogacy. I had to trust that the agency had screened her thoroughly and competently. I also had to hope that I could overcome my snobbery, be tolerant, and like or grow to like someone whose socio-economic background and education are so different from my own. With the encouragement and reassurance of Roger and our counselor, we arranged our first meeting with Donna and Steve.

Roger and I flew down to southern California the night before we were to meet Donna, Steve, and the counselor for lunch. I spent the next morning getting sick to my stomach because I was so nervous about meeting Donna. When we arrived at the restaurant, Donna and Steve were sitting at a table on the terrace waiting for us. As soon as we approached them Donna hugged me and everyone seemed instantly relieved. Months later Donna told me that I had looked quite pale and terrified at that first encounter. Susan, the counselor met us a few minutes later and, after giving us some guidelines and introducing everyone, left us to our own devices. The lunch went smoothly, and everyone got along well. We talked about our jobs, hobbies, travel, and families. It was like being on a blind date. We even exchanged phone numbers and promised to be in touch soon. Donna and Steve then invited us back to their home nearby to meet their children and see their house. Their home was perfectly nice and their family, delightful and healthy. We were impressed at how well they managed raising four young children. Basically, none of my fears were realized; the walls of their home weren't covered with crucifixes or Biblical verses; the house was clean and organized; the kids seemed happy and well taken care of; and Donna and Steve appeared to get along well and be perfectly sane and pleasant. The next day, Roger and I met Donna and her oldest child for lunch and a walk, and again, everyone got on well and had a fine time.

Our fears allayed, Roger and I returned home ready to begin the surrogacy process with Donna. We felt comfortable with her and fairly confident that the relationship could work and that Donna would be a trustworthy, conscientious gestational surrogate. She had already told us that she wanted to work with us. So, we contacted the agency, had the contracts drafted, completed all of the paperwork, set up a trust for Donna that would be administered by the agency to reimburse her and pay her, arranged consultations at the fertility center we would be using, and all in all, got the process underway. In retrospect, compared to what awaited us, this part of the process was easy and painless. However, it was merely the beginning. This phase involved weeks of phone calls, emails, faxes, travel arrangements, and mountains of paperwork all amounting to what was to become a part-time occupation and full-time preoccupation.

## Chapter 6

After a bit of research and many phone calls, we decided to use a fertility clinic in Orange County. The clinic came highly recommended from the surrogacy agency, and it was the most convenient one for Donna. Our surrogate had an initial consultation with one of the doctors at the clinic, whom she found affable, so after researching him a bit, Roger and I flew down to Orange County to meet him as well. The Orange County IVF clinic was in a high rise medical office building adjacent to a hospital. After a prolonged wait in a nicely appointed waiting room, which we would soon learn was reserved for people waiting for consultations, and not actual patients, we met with Dr. P., who was in fact friendly and had a dry sense of humor. After reviewing our medical records and listening to our story, Dr. P. familiarly said, "You know that you can't replace the babies you lost." Evidently, this was a line that both perinatologists and infertility specialists learned in their residencies. Roger and I nodded wearily. Dr. P. explained the IVF procedures to us in some detail, and believed that we were promising candidates. I then asked Dr. P. if there was evidence that IVF caused long-term damage. He said no, that babies born from IVF appeared to be healthy and normal. However, he did not realize that I was asking about myself. I never got a clear answer from him.

Coordinating IVF with an egg donor (me) and a surrogate involved a fairly complex set of procedures and logistics. Once Donna and I passed thorough extensive medical screenings and got our periods we could begin the process. A few days after menstruating we would each begin taking birth control pills for a few weeks. Next we and our husbands had to take a regimen of antibiotics to kill any lurking infections. After being on the pill, Donna and I, at different times, began injecting ourselves with a drug called Lupron, which regulates the pituitary gland and, in turn, decreases the production of estrogen and progesterone, essentially putting us into a menopause-like state. Presumably this is so that we can be stimulated later with various hormones to produce eggs, in my case, or a thick uterine lining for pregnancy, in Donna's case. Essentially, the fertility doctor suppresses a woman's reproductive system so that he can more accurately control it in the second phase of the IVF process. Once Donna and I were ready to start taking the pill, we had to visit the clinic for injection lessons with Dr. P.'s nurse. Armed with needles and various vials, we were ready to begin our first round of IVF.

For many women contemplating IVF or about to undergo it, daily injections are the biggest fear and impediment. Under most IVF protocols, it is necessary to inject oneself or be injected at least twice a day over the course of a few weeks. From my own experience and from those of friends who underwent IVF, the shots are a relatively minor inconvenience compared to the more incapacitating side effects and aspects of the fertility treatments. It is hard for me to imagine how anyone can work full time and at full function while undergoing this treatment. For the duration of the protocol, IVF took over my life.

The IVF regimen began with taking birth control pills for a couple of weeks. Millions of women take birth control pills and have few if any unpleasant side effects. However, almost as soon as I began taking the pill I felt queasy and experienced gastro-intestinal discomfort and diarrhea. According to Dr. M., this is not uncommon during the first few weeks of taking the pill. But I took the pill for only a few weeks, so I never adapted to it. To compound the problem, I had to take antibiotics for five days while on the pill. And this was supposed to be the easy part of the protocol.

Towards the end of my bout with the pill, I had to begin injecting myself daily with Lupron, the estrogen and progesterone suppressant. The injections themselves were easy to administer since the needles were small and the drug fairly simple to upload into the needle, much like the older style of insulin shots. However, the side effects of Lupron were utterly insidious. It was like undergoing PMS one hundred fold. I was overcome by mood swings ranging from deep depression to sheer rage that terrified me and made me almost unrecognizable to Roger. It was as if I were possessed. I have never felt so out of control and alienated from myself. When Roger returned home from work each evening he tentatively approached me, probably fearing for his life, and asked if I was "Lupronius." He meant this coinage to be a proper noun, referring to the tyrannical Roman emperor, Lupronius. I assumed that he was using the word as an adjective, asking me if I was "lupronious," as in "Are you in a lupronious or friendly mood today?" Either way, I was undoubtedly in a state and to be avoided. After about a week on Lupron I began to have unbearable headaches, comparable to migraines. I felt too incapacitated to drive and would have to lie down in a dark room pressing a hot washcloth on my temples. Nothing would eradicate the headaches; at best, I could dull them for a few hours by takng over-the-counter pain killers. Apparently, the headaches are a common effect of the drug and showed that it was in fact lowering my estrogen levels. This experience did not bode well for menopause, though menopause, for better or worse, isn't a concentrated two week event.

*The Maternity Labyrinth*

After a couple of weeks of Lupron, my estrogen levels were deemed to be sufficiently lowered, and I was certifiably insane, I began the ovary stimulation phase. In addition to a lower daily dose of Lupron, I now had to add two more injections of gonadotropins. My headaches and moodiness disappeared almost as soon as I began taking them. In this round of IVF, I was prescribed two different kinds of gonadotropins. Each came in powder form and had to be mixed with sterile water before being absorbed into the syringe and injected. I had heard rumors about the nuisance of "mixing" IVF medications and never understood them. Now I had the pleasure of doing it myself. Using a long, scary needle, I first took up a specified amount of water into the syringe. I then had to eject the water into a vial of the powdered medicine. Then I needed to suck up this mixture back into the syringe. I repeated this procedure using a few vials. When I was done mixing and reabsorbing the required amount, I had to change the needle head so that I wouldn't then stab myself with a preposterously long and wide needle that looked like a very dangerous turkey baster. Changing the needle head or taking off the needle cap didn't always run smoothly. I poked myself in the finger a number of times when one of them got stuck or was too tightly secured. The second drug came in all-glass, bullet-shaped, capless vials, meaning that I had to snap off the glass tip and try to avoid cutting my hand while breaking the glass tips or on the jagged rims. This drug also needed to be mixed. Unlike giving myself Lupron, which I still had to do, preparing and injecting the gonadotropins took quite a bit of time and caused a great deal of frustration. I simply don't have the patience or temperament of a chemist to enjoy such experiments.

I found the side effects of the stimulating hormones less onerous than those of Lupron. My abdomen became slightly distended as my ovaries filled with many eggs, and as a result, it was a bit uncomfortable to walk and sit. I was forbidden to do any vigorous exercise and didn't really feel up to it anyway. By this time in the IVF process, I had also acquired countless needle marks and bruises on my thighs and abdomen. According to Dr. P.'s nurse, my estrogen levels were "through the roof," and Dr. P. had some concern about over stimulating me, which could cause my body to fill with fluid after the egg retrieval and lead to other complications. At that point, however, I didn't feel too bad. From my perspective, this stage was certainly preferable to my Lupron-induced psychosis.

During this entire time Donna and I talked regularly on the phone and compared notes about our experiences. She too had Lupron-related headaches and crankiness, but managed to escape the nausea from the pill. Instead of taking gonadotropins or another drug that required mixing,

Donna in addition to taking various pills, had to be injected with various viscous medications, among them progesterone, to build up her uterine lining and prepare her for pregnancy. The needles for these injections were large and had to be administered by her husband, Steve. The huge needles and the oily medicines caused bruising and hard spots on the injection sites. But Donna never complained and always maintained her optimism and sense of humor. It's possible that Donna was less sensitive than I, especially to the Lupron. The various people I've talked to who have undergone IVF have all had different reactions in varying degrees to the drugs. Many of my friends and even Dr. M. have described me as stoic. I don't believe that I've exaggerated my response to the Lupron, and I tried my best to cope with its effects. It is possible that my reaction to it was more intense than Donna's not only because I'm more sensitive to it physically, but also because I was more invested in the entire IVF and baby-making process emotionally. I had experienced loss and knew that things could go wrong. I could manage to pull off stoicism in public, but in private, I was Lupronius the Great.

Throughout the course of my IVF regimen, I was monitored by a local fertility clinic. The staff and doctors in this clinic were extraordinarily kind and helpful, in contrast to what I would soon discover about the Orange County clinic. At the fertility center near my house, I never had to wait for any procedure more than a few minutes. The nurses who drew my blood seemed to be concerned about my well-being and the outcome of the IVF. The doctors were attentive, listened, and answered any questions I had. I never felt rushed or dismissed. After examining me one doctor said "Thank you for all you do." Admittedly, I was not saving the world, but I was grateful that in his own way he could acknowledge that IVF was emotionally and physically taxing. Depending on what stage of the process I was in, I had to have blood tests to determine my hormone levels and ultrasounds to count and measure my eggs once or twice a week. I have never been particularly squeamish about needles, but after a few weeks of multiple daily injections and bi-weekly blood draws, I came to loathe them. My arms were now also covered in bruises from the needles, collapsed veins, and botched attempts at drawing my blood. The ultrasounds monitored egg follicles and egg development. I was quite productive; I had grown approximately twenty-two eggs! Apparently that was quite impressive for a woman my age. The results were regularly faxed to Dr. P.'s office in Orange County, and he adjusted my dosages accordingly. So far, things were going even better than anticipated.

A few days before the scheduled egg retrieval, Roger and I drove down to southern California. Since we would be down there for over a week, we thought it would be easier to have our own car. I also didn't want to deal with dragging my swollen abdomen and luggage through the airport and argue with security about my stash of medications and needles. The day after we arrived in Orange County I would be examined by Dr. P. Two days later my eggs would be removed. After a few days of recovery for me and development time for the fertilized eggs, the embryos would then be transferred to Donna. Donna would then have to spend three days on bed rest in a hotel room. Since she has four little children running around she felt that she couldn't possibly maintain bed rest while at home. We decided to keep Donna company at the hotel while she was confined. By that time I was likely to feel well and Donna could go home and keep her fingers crossed for two weeks until her pregnancy test.

While waiting for my pre-retrieval exam with Dr. P., I got my first inkling that the Orange County fertility center was a big IVF factory. I and many other women and their partners had to wait for ages in a waiting area with insufficient seating before we were seen. I was stunned by the sheer number of people who were patients at that clinic. Could this many women in one county all be infertile? When I was finally examined by Dr. P., I felt rushed and discouraged from asking questions even though he was perfectly pleasant. Basically, he was very busy and had little time to focus on each individual patient. My concerns about the fertility center were confirmed by my future experiences there.

Exactly thirty-six hours before my scheduled egg retrieval, Roger had to inject me in the rear end with hCG (human chorionic gonadotropin), which triggers ovulation. This drug also requires mixing and involves two large needles, one for mixing and one for injecting. Roger managed to poke himself in the finger while changing the needle head. Fortunately, he never showed any signs of ovulating. The nurse had given Roger shooting lessons and drawn a target on my behind so that Roger could inject me in the right spot and avoid hitting my sciatic nerve. Despite his nervousness, he did a fine job, and I went to bed with an appropriately sore butt but generally unscathed.

A day and a half later we were back in Dr. P.'s office waiting for ages to have the egg retrieval. It seemed odd to me that I could be kept waiting so long when the hCG injection had to be timed so precisely. The eggs needed to be aspirated when they were loosened but before they were released. Evidently there was some flexibility here. While I was kept waiting, Roger had to go off to a private room to make his sperm donation. He had plenty of time. In the egg retrieval procedure, a doctor puts a needle through the vaginal wall and aspirates the eggs in each ovary. I would be under anesthesia (twilight sleep) during the procedure. I was at last brought in to the operating room, prepped, and anesthetized. It struck me as a bit strange that a radio station playing pop music of the seventies was on and that the nurses and anesthesiologist were chatting with each other as if I weren't in the room. Dr. P. wasn't there yet and would make his grand entrance when I was unconscious. The atmosphere seemed dream like, as if they were having a party to which I was not invited. About an hour later, after the procedure, I was roused and given a little while to revive. Dr. P. came in briefly to let me know that he had retrieved twenty-two mature eggs. He noted that this was quite an accomplishment for a woman of my advanced years. This was just one of his numerous comments about my age. To a fertility doctor, anyone over thirty-five is old and over forty, on her death bed. I had just turned forty. It didn't seem to matter to him, or perhaps he didn't remember that I was using this clinic because of my need for a gestational surrogate and not to remedy infertility.

After the retrieval, Roger ushered me in my woozy state out of the office with instructions to make sure that I remain in bed the rest of the day, take pain killers to alleviate cramping, and drink plenty of fluids. The recovery wasn't that bad. I had mild cramping and was sleepy and bloated but managed to avoid hyperstimulation syndrome. After a few days, I felt pretty good. The day after the retrieval the nurse called to let us know that seventeen of the twenty-two eggs fertilized. After two more days they could determine how well the embryos were developing and which were worthy of implanting or freezing. The plan was that Roger and I would meet Donna and Steve at Dr. P.'s office to decide, with Dr. P.'s guidance, how many embryos to transfer. If everyone was prepared, Donna's lining was sufficiently thick, and the embryos were ready to go, the transfer would take place.

On the third day we all congregated in the waiting area of the clinic where we had quite a bit of time to chat and get to know each other even better. When we were finally called in to the examination room, Dr. P. sat down with us and showed us photos of our embryos. Twelve of the seventeen embryos had continued to develop and of those, approximately five to seven had a sufficient number of cells and little fragmentation. Dr. P. suggested that he transfer five embryos, explaining that even though my egg production was plentiful, I was forty years old and therefore my eggs were likely to produce some unviable embryos with chromosomal abnormalities. He felt that it was highly improbable that more than one embryo would stick and thought that our odds of having a pregnancy were much higher transferring five than putting in two or three. He found it irrelevant that

I had had no problem conceiving a mere year and a half earlier and that neither of my fetuses had genetic abnormalities. Dr. P. estimated that we had a fifty percent chance of having a positive pregnancy. That statistic sounded awfully high to me, especially after having read many articles that mentioned average success rates of thirty percent using IVF. Perhaps he was trying to be optimistic and encouraging. Maybe he was impressed by my prolific egg production. We nervously agreed to transfer five embryos into Donna's uterus. Before Roger and I left the room and Dr. P. conducted the procedure he asserted enthusiastically, "We're going to make a baby." We certainly hoped so.

The transfer, which consisted of using some kind of catheter through which the embryos were placed in Donna's uterus, was quick and painless, according to Donna. After the procedure Donna had to remain horizontal on the exam table for about half an hour. When she had completed her reclining period, we all returned to the hotel so that Donna could relax for a few days. Although everyone was rather anxious, we had a pleasant time chatting, watching movies and TV, and eating food from take-out and room service. Over the course of those three days, Donna, Steve, Roger, and I got to know each other better. The more time I spent with Donna, the more I trusted her and felt comfortable that she would be carrying our baby.

After Donna's three days of confinement in a hotel and our week plus stay in the *Twilight Zone* of Orange County, we all returned to our respective homes to wait. Throughout the two-week waiting period, Donna kept me posted about any possible pregnancy symptoms. She claimed to feel tired and queasy. This gave me hope, but I knew to be cautious and not assume too much. Donna had been told not to take a home pregnancy test. The surrogacy agency wanted to make sure that she was not responsible for being the bearer of good or bad tidings and that a pregnancy be confirmed by a doctor. I spent the day of Donna's Beta test staring at my cell phone. That afternoon Dr. P.'s nurse called with the disappointing news that Donna was not pregnant. Needless to say, we were upset. Although we knew the statistics about IVF success rates, we were led to believe that our chances were pretty good. When I had agreed to try IVF, I told myself that I would play the odds if I had to, namely try it up to three times, since there was a thirty-something percent chance of getting pregnant each time. Now knowing what it was like to go through a round of IVF, I was dreading doing it ever again, let alone a third time.

We had to wait about two months for Donna's and my cycles to return back to normal before we could begin round two of IVF. I'm not sure which is worse, anticipating an unknown as I did with round one, or dreading a known, which constituted the waiting period before round two. I spent those few weeks making arrangements with the fertility center, signing more contracts, and making travel plans again to Orange County. I thought about different ways to make this next go of IVF less unpleasant. One friend, who went through three rounds of IVF and had a rough time of it, suggested that I try acupuncture. Had almost anyone else recommended it, I would have scoffed, but this friend is a scientist, a skeptic, and understood my own skepticism. So I listened. She claimed that acupuncture helped her relax and took some of the edge off of the unpleasant side effects of IVF. She gave me the name of the person she used who had been recommended by her fertility doctor. After checking with my own doctor, I decided to give it a try. I had nothing to lose; if I found it unpleasant, I could quit. Perhaps it would help to alleviate the horrible Lupron headaches or calm me so that I wouldn't be as cranky.

As soon as I started taking the birth control pill again, I called the acupuncturist and set up an appointment for a consultation. His office was in a very modest apartment building, and his waiting room reeked of medicinal-smelling herbs. The waiting area consisted of a few chairs and a desk and was adjacent to a long room filled with beds that were separated by curtains. The calm and gentle acupuncturist, Dr. Z., had a medical degree from China and was certified by the state of California. He asked me questions about my general health and about my fertility and IVF history. His questions indicated that he was well informed about the IVF process. He made no promises and used no silly jargon but said that he would focus on alleviating my headaches, relaxing me, and increasing blood flow. He explained a bit how acupuncture works and suggested that I see him once or twice a week. I couldn't believe that I was agreeing to undergo acupuncture. I was desperate and would try pretty much anything that wasn't harmful.

The following week when I appeared at my first acupuncture session, Dr. Z. greeted me and conducted me to one of the tables. I was told to take off my shoes and lie down face up. The curtains were drawn around one of the other tables at the end of the row, which I figured was occupied by someone who was quietly relaxing while all needled up. The other beds were uninhabited. Dr. Z. then took out a bunch of individually wrapped needles and alcohol pads. He explained where he'd be sticking the needles and told me that once they were in I should relax or sleep. He would remove them in about half an hour or so. Dr. Z. put small, very thin needles in the tops of my feet, the fronts of my calves, hands, and forehead. It stung a bit when he put in the needles, but after a few seconds I no longer noticed them. He then closed the curtains surrounding my bed and left me to rest. While I was attempting to relax a man walked in and was guided to the table next to mine. He spoke in a loud, assertive voice, which was jarring on its own and particularly in contrast to that of Dr. Z. After the obtrusive man was needled, Dr. Z. closed his curtain and returned to his desk. Seconds later, the man began to snore with loud, annoying, rasping and snorting sounds. We were only a few feet apart, separated by a mere curtain. There was no way I could sleep or relax having to listen to him. After a while, Dr. Z. returned to remove my needles. I can't say that I felt particularly at peace with the world, but I figured I'd give it another try. I made sure to schedule my next session at a different time so that I could avoid the snorer.

I continued to get acupuncture treatments once or twice a week for the remainder of that IVF cycle. When there was no one else snoring or talking in one of the neighboring beds, I could usually relax and even doze off for a bit. Roger claimed that I seemed calmer and less volatile when I returned from acupuncture, especially while on Lupron. I didn't feel much calmer, though perhaps a bit fuzzy after I left, but I attributed that to having had nap time in the middle of the day. One of my acupuncture sessions was deliberately scheduled during the horrid headache stage of IVF. Dr. Z. asked me where my head hurt, and I indicated over my right eye. He placed some needles, I guess strategically, on the top of my left foot. After a few minutes it felt as if the tension was draining from over my right eye. By the time the session was over, my headache was just about gone. I remained headache free for the rest of the day. It did return the next afternoon, but I was grateful for the twenty-four hour reprieve. Acupuncture worked better than Advil, so I stuck with it and became a believer.

My experience throughout the second round of IVF was very similar to that of my first bout. Again, I grew many eggs, about the same number, and I was moody and uncomfortable. Besides the acupuncture, another improvement in this round was that I no longer had to mix the gonadotropins. I was now taking only one kind of stimulating hormone which came in a pre-mixed pen that was easy to inject and required little preparation. I was relieved to be excused from IVF chemistry lab. The only irritation of using the pen was that it emitted a creepy clicking sound when the medicine was injected and it left an odd smell of alcohol and plastic which I could almost taste. It was still an improvement over the days of snapping glass vials and ineptly mixing various formulas and poking myself in the wrong places.

After a few weeks of the all-consuming IVF drug phase, Roger and I drove down to Orange County again for the retrieval and transfer. Everything was pretty much the same—the extraordinary traffic driving through LA, the nice hotel that I now thought of as a convalescent home, the long waits at the fertility center, the hCG shot administered by Roger in the hotel bathroom, and entertaining Donna while she was resting in her hotel room. This round, good hen that I was, I produced twenty-three eggs. Of those, eighteen fertilized and six looked good enough to transfer. We all gasped when Dr. P. recommended transferring six embryos. But he argued, yet again, that because of my age and because the last transfer failed, he thought he should be aggressive. He still contended it was unlikely that Donna would become pregnant with multiples but was optimistic that we would have a pregnancy. So he prevailed, and we acquiesced.

After a few days of recovering from the egg retrieval and staying with Donna while she was on bed rest in the hotel, we did the long drive home again and began the wait. The Beta test was scheduled for the day before Thanksgiving, so we would either have much to be thankful for or bitter about. Roger and I usually spend the holiday in New York with my parents. Since we did not want to be on an airplane and unavailable the day we found out the news and preferred to be home if the news was bad, we decided to host Thanksgiving and invited my parents and Roger's mother. Clearly, we were not of sound minds when we made this decision. My parents were delighted to come to California and made plans immediately. Roger's mother, who no longer traveled much, was non-committal and less enthusiastic. At the last minute, she decided to attend. I had assumed that she would not. The idea of her and my parents in close contact over the course of a few days was horrifying. The combination of my liberal, Jewish, New Yorker parents with Roger's conservative, Protestant, Oklahoman mother would cause a spontaneous combustion at the Thanksgiving table. My hormonally-induced lunacy and anxiety about the outcome of this round of IVF weren't helping me cope with this predicament that I had created.

In the days preceding Thanksgiving I shopped and cooked and tried to distract myself as much as possible. It turned out that our guests would overlap for only two full days. My parents arrived on Sunday and left on Friday, while Roger's mother arrived Tuesday night and left on Sunday. Everyone would be with us on that tension-filled Wednesday. Roger would be at work half that day; my parents would drop by around noon, and Roger's mother would appear a little later in the afternoon. At about noon, while I was preparing the hazelnut stuffing, my cell phone, the phone on which I received all fertility and maternity-related calls, rang. I could tell the minute I heard Dr. P.'s nurse's tone that it was bad news. She had the serious, I'm-so-sorry timbre to her voice. It was in fact disappointing news: no pregnancy. This time I was crushed and shocked. While I was on the phone with the nurse, my parents arrived. They took one look at me, figured out what was up, and tactfully said that they would go get lunch and return in a little while. I called Roger at work immediately. He was as stunned as I was. He said that he'd be home in a little while. Soon after, Roger called to tell me that while backing out, he accidentally hit someone's car in the parking lot of his office building because he was so distracted and upset. My parents then returned. Roger's mother arrived before Roger got home, and upon entering immediately asked, "Any news yet?" I believe that my parents may have intervened. All I remember beyond the fact that I didn't slug her, was that I started chopping hazelnuts with a hammer. They were finely crushed.

Much to my astonishment, Thanksgiving dinner went smoothly. The parents behaved well enough and got along. Everyone tried to make pleasant chit chat. Nonetheless, my already low tolerance for Roger's mother reached its nadir that week. She had an uncanny way of saying precisely the wrong thing at the wrong time. She would spontaneously ask questions about the IVF process or second-guess the doctors, or she would falsely comfort us with such comments as "I know it will work next time." My attitude was how does she know? My belief in the powers of IVF and in everyone's predictions was waning by the minute. After a few more fraught days all the guests departed and Roger and I were left alone to recover from them and to figure out what to do next.

That Monday I spoke to our counselor from the surrogacy agency, who was helpful and encouraging. She mentioned that it takes two to three tries of IVF for most of their clients. She also suggested that we call Dr. P. to see if he had any insights or advice. I called Dr. P.'s office and asked to speak to him or be connected to his voice mail. In an accusatory tone, the receptionist, who seemed to feel that her main role was to keep infiltrators away, asked why I was calling and made it clear that I could not speak to Dr. P. without scheduling a phone conference with him. In order to do so, I would have to call his nurse. So I called his nurse and scheduled a phone call with him for one week later. He would call me at an appointed time.

One week later Dr. P. called at the designated hour. He did not have an answer for why the IVF did not work other than blaming me and my ancient eggs. When I asked him if it was possible that there was a problem with Donna or Roger, he said that it was very unlikely. Usually embryos aren't viable because of the donor's eggs. Besides, Donna had a "great uterus," her hormone levels were just right, and her uterine lining was perfect. She also had a fine track record with her own pregnancies. When I bluntly asked him if we were crazy to continue with this process, he said absolutely not.

According to Dr. P., I responded well to the protocol and produced large quantities of eggs. By no means was my case hopeless. I tried to squelch my terribly skeptical thought that Dr. P. couldn't be trusted since he had nothing to lose and a great deal of money to gain from our repeated attempts of IVF. But it was hard to swallow that a doctor could be so insidiously mercenary and heartless as to take advantage of us like that. I had to hope that he had our best interests in mind and was being fair and honest. I've never been wholly convinced of either argument.

So we plugged on and worked on scheduling the third, and as far as I was concerned, the last round of IVF. I called Dr. P.'s nurse to let her know that we wanted to try another round of IVF and to get the process started again. In all of my previous interactions with Dr. P.'s nurse, and there were many, she had been kind, reliable, clear, organized, well-informed, compassionate, and helpful. For some strange reason, that day she began to lecture me about the dangers of IVF and the long-term risks, like uterine cancer, of doing it many times. I reminded her that I'd undergone the procedure only twice. Evidently she was confusing me with another patient who was about to try round seven. I was also outraged that now I was being warned about the possibilities of developing uterine cancer in the future. Why didn't Dr. P. say anything about this when I asked him in our initial consultation? In the many contracts I signed I acknowledged various warnings about ovarian hyperstimulation and bad reactions to anesthesia, but nothing about IVF-induced cancer. It turns out that the findings about long-term effects of IVF are controversial and not conclusive. Nonetheless, I was completely unnerved by the nurse's faux pas, distrustful of Dr. P., and if possible, even less enthusiastic about proceeding to round three.

Once again I devoted a great deal of time and thought to arranging this IVF stint. The all-too familiar contracts, phone calls, blood tests, hotel reservations, and coordinating of Donna's and my schedules, cycles, and lives made me into my own personal assistant. The hotel we usually stayed at was fully booked. Despite the fine service and accommodations of the hotel, I was relieved to stay elsewhere. That hotel had nothing but bad associations for me: sickness, confinement, and failure. My attitude towards Orange County, which was not great to begin with, was equally negative. I was tired of the ubiquitous malls and the inappropriately green grass in a desert region. I was sick of being confined to a hotel room for a week, and I was exhausted from the eight hour car rides along the mind-numbing, fast-food littered interstate freeway. My outlook towards this third try was complicated. I was not optimistic but felt that everything was riding on the outcome of this protocol. It was unlikely that I'd undergo IVF again after this. If it didn't work, Roger and I would have to rethink our options and come up with a new plan. I was also somewhat relieved or resigned, since I believed that at least we'd have an answer one way or another after this round, and I wouldn't have to put myself through this form of torture again. What was so maddening was that we had no good explanation as to why IVF hadn't worked so far. It was difficult to determine when to give up since there was nothing or no one to blame for the failure. Since everything about this experience turned out to be a giant gamble, we figured that we'd just play the odds.

Round three proceeded, much like rounds one and two. Donna and I were very consistent in our responses to the medications. I returned to Dr. Z. for acupuncture treatments hoping that he could alleviate my discomfort and headaches again. Unfortunately, Dr. Z. was unable to perform any headache-eliminating miracles this time, and I became as disillusioned with Eastern treatments as I had already become with Western medicine. In fact, this time, I found acupuncture to be little more than a nuisance. I didn't find it relaxing to lie on a bed while listening to my neighbor snoring or talking. I also didn't relish the opportunity to be poked with any extra needles. My self-inflicted injections were more than enough.

This round my egg production reached a personal best—over thirty! Dr. P. was slightly more aggressive this time with my doses of gonadotropins, perhaps figuring that he may as well harvest as many eggs as possible since I wasn't going to keep doing this indefinitely. Except for ruining my associations with a different perfectly nice hotel, everything else about our visit to Orange County, the retrieval, and the transfer was pretty much the same as ever. As always, over seventy percent of my eggs successfully fertilized. Dr. P. now wanted to transfer seven embryos to Donna. Everyone, including the nurse, looked alarmed. Apparently that would set a new record for Dr. P. He contended that it hadn't worked so far, and he still believed that there was only a very small chance of having a twin pregnancy and next to no chance of more than that. So in the mere few minutes that we had to make a decision, based on little more than Dr. P.'s counsel and a bit of previous research, we approved the transfer of seven embryos to Donna's womb. It wasn't comforting to imagine that we might be cited in the annals of reproductive medicine.

A little less than two weeks later I received a package in the mail from Donna that included a stuffed bear that was dressed like a baby and holding a bottle. Given my pessimism and cynicism I was rather mystified by the gift. Donna's pregnancy test wasn't scheduled for another two days. It seemed a bit presumptuous of her to assume that she'd be pregnant. I also am not a big fan of stuffed animals for myself. Later that day Donna called and asked if I had received the package. I said yes and tried to sound enthusiastic about the cuteness of the bear. She replied, "and?," but I didn't know what she was driving at. After some confusion Donna asked if I'd heard her message. Apparently, I was supposed to press on one of the bear's paws to hear a recorded message. So I pressed the paw and heard Donna's voice saying, "Congratulations! You're having a baby!" After I got over my confusion and amazement, Donna explained that she took the pregnancy test a few days early because she was nauseated and tired. Dr. P.'s nurse gave her permission to be the first to let me know, and she would call me later to confirm the pregnancy. We had become so accustomed to disappointment that it took a while to believe and allow ourselves to feel happy about this first bit of encouraging news.

Two weeks later, Roger and I flew down to Orange County for the first ultrasound. We would find out if the embryo had a heartbeat and if we were expecting one or more babies. Donna's weekly blood tests indicated high hormone levels, which suggested that she might be carrying multiples. We met Donna once again in the waiting room for the usual extended wait to see Dr. P. Then we were brought into the exam room where Donna was prepped, and we waited in anticipation for Dr. P. to arrive and perform the ultrasound. Dr. P. entered the room, we all made chit chat, and he began the ultrasound. All eyes were on the monitor, which would show what was going on inside Donna's uterus. I glanced at the monitor and thought that I saw a few blobs. I then looked at Dr. P. I will never forget the expression on his face, an unsettled, what-have I done look. He seemed horrified because there were four distinct embryos with heartbeats. Yes. We were expecting quadruplets. Everyone was stunned, and no one was particularly delighted by this unanticipated turn of events. Dr. P. explained that in all of his years of practice he had never seen a forty-year old who had two failed rounds of IVF then produce a quadruplet pregnancy. He said that it was very unlikely that all four would make it to the end of the first trimester, which might be a blessing since carrying four babies is extremely dangerous for the carrier and the babies. He also explained that miscarrying one or more embryos could cause a domino-like effect and endanger the entire pregnancy. Dr. P. recommended reducing the pregnancy to two or three but advised waiting before making a decision, since nature was likely to take its course.

This was complete madness. Here we'd been worried about having one baby and now we were faced with a terrible medical and moral dilemma of what to do about quadruplets. We were willing to reduce if necessary but were very disturbed by the idea. Here we'd tried so hard to get pregnant and now we were contemplating aborting. Reducing a pregnancy can also endanger the other embryos. Besides, how does one decide which embryo to eliminate? The smallest, sickliest looking one? Does one then have amniocentesis or CVS to help make such a decision? I felt like I was participating in a freakish science experiment. I would have to make impossible decisions that I did not want to make.

By now, I was convinced that I was a statistical anomaly when it came to pregnancy. From my first pregnancy to this most recent fiasco, I defied every prediction and probability. I was one of the one to two percent of women who have an incompetent cervix; I was in the tenth percentile for whom bed rest and cerclage do not work; I appeared to be quite fertile, producing an unusually large number of eggs for a forty-year old; despite that, I had failed to produce a pregnancy in two rounds of IVF; finally, with a less than one percent chance, I produced a quadruplet pregnancy. By this point, I believed none of the predictions that Dr. P. or any other fertility specialist, perinatologist, or obstetrician made. And there was nothing I could do about our situation. We simply had to wait until the next week and the next ultrasound to see how things developed.

In the meantime, Donna was advised to go on bed rest. Frankly, I never saw much justification for this. Perhaps I had taken on Dr. D.'s attitude. It seemed to me that if Donna was going to miscarry in the first trimester, there was little to be done to stop it. As Dr. P. said, it might be for the best anyway. Also, this meant that Donna needed to find a full-time babysitter and helper to cook and clean. None of us had anticipated this situation. The whole point of working with a surrogate was to avoid a high-risk pregnancy. Now we were no better off that we had been when I was pregnant and on bed rest.

Over the weekend Donna started bleeding, which we all assumed was a miscarriage. We had to wait a few days before the next ultrasound to determine how many miscarried. The next ultrasound was hard to read. Dr. P. was fairly certain that there were now two remaining embryos, but there was so much tissue and blood in Donna's uterus that it was hard to determine for sure. So Dr. P. sent us to see a perinatologist who worked in the adjacent medical center and who possessed particularly sensitive and sophisticated ultrasound equipment. Donna, who was supposed to be on bed rest, and I trudged over to the perinatologist's office. Sure enough, there were two surviving embryos which had good heartbeats and seemed to be growing properly. He explained, however, that the pregnancy was still at high risk because of clotting, and circulating hormones and tissue from the lost embryos. He advised that Donna remain on bed rest and return the following week.

At the next ultrasound we were down to one. The one remaining embryo had a strong heartbeat, a nicely developed sac, was growing appropriately, and was well situated near the fundus. Donna was disappointed because she was excited about carrying twins for us and had carried her own successfully, but Roger and I were perfectly content with a singleton. The pregnancy was less risky. If Donna got through the rest of the first trimester, we might actually be able to relax a bit and assume that the rest of the pregnancy would be normal. In the meanwhile, Donna was told to remain on bed rest and return for another ultrasound.

Once again, I flew down to Orange County for another ultrasound. Donna continued to feel queasy and tired and was gaining weight. Her hormone levels were also increasing properly. When Dr. P. looked at the ultrasound monitor he looked disturbed and announced that he didn't see a heartbeat in the remaining embryo. He recommended that we visit the perinatologist again in the next building to double check. It didn't look promising. Off we went to the office of high tech equipment to get more bad news. And then there were none. There was in fact no heartbeat. The embryo must have died a few days earlier since it was measuring eight weeks and three days, and Donna was now over nine weeks pregnant. Donna burst into tears. I remained my usual stoic self. Loss and disappointment were commonplace for me by this point. I expected them. After talking to the technician and doctor we returned to Dr. P.'s office to consult with him and confirm the news. Dr. P. actually sat down and talked with us for a while. His assumption, again, was that the embryos probably weren't viable because of my aged eggs. Yes. It was my fault. It was possible that there was a domino effect or that some of the embryos didn't attach properly. He wasn't certain. He recommended that Donna have a D and C to make sure that all of the tissue was removed properly. He wanted to test the tissue to see if he could determine if there were genetic problems in the embryos but was fairly certain that he couldn't, given the number of embryos and what a mess it was in Donna's uterus. But he'd try. He had no real answers for us. Roger and I wouldn't have to make any difficult decisions about reduction after all.

The big question was what to do next. I had vowed that I wouldn't undergo more than three rounds of IVF, and I wasn't sure that I could handle another one. Roger wasn't particularly enthusiastic about adoption. We could try using an egg donor, but I was strongly opposed to it and still wasn't convinced that my eggs were faulty. The fact that I had produced so many eggs each time and that Donna had gotten pregnant this last round were encouraging signs. Dr. P. still didn't think it was hopeless. Donna had the D and C, but Dr. P. was unable to test the tissue. While Donna recovered from the procedure and her body returned to normal, Roger and I had some time to think about our next move. After much discussion and fretting, I agreed to try one last round of IVF. My attitude was poor; I was doing it grudgingly. At the time it still seemed preferable to our other options.

While we were waiting and stewing about the upcoming cycle, I called a friend who had recently adopted a child in the United States. I was hoping to learn a bit more about domestic adoption and hear an encouraging story that I could share with Roger. My friend and her husband had adopted a baby boy a few months earlier. She was deliriously happy. Her son was healthy and thriving, and she was enjoying motherhood. I believe that she thought she was giving me a pep talk about adopting, but after I got off the phone with her I lost interest in domestic adoption. Even though she received custody of her son immediately after he was born, the adoption still hadn't been finalized because there is a six month waiting period in her state, during which time the birth mother can change her mind and take back the baby. My friend had also described, in detail, the logistics of adopting, including the various forms and questionnaires they filled out. She admitted to agreeing to adopt the child of a woman who smoked throughout her pregnancy. My friend explained that if she had ruled out smoking, drinking, and drug use, she never would have gotten a baby. So she figured that smoking was slightly less harmful than the others and checked off that box. Her story ended happily, but I was not comforted by it. I suppose that people could find all sorts of problems with surrogacy. I had certainly experienced numerous disappointments. For me, however, it was important to know that the woman carrying my baby, Donna, was not abusing her body or harming the developing baby while pregnant and would have no claims on the baby once it was born. Anyone who wants to have a child and is unable to produce one naturally on her own ends up making compromises and taking risks. I was still willing to gamble on surrogacy.

After a two month recovery period, Donna and I began round four of IVF. The medications, symptoms, egg production, and everything else were all pretty much the same as they had been. I chose to forego acupuncture this time. It hadn't been all that helpful and I didn't need any extraneous injections. The one difference in our approach this round was that we would do PGD (preimplantation genetic diagnosis) on the embryos. In this procedure, the embryologist removes one cell from each three-day old embryo and tests it to determine a variety of genetic disorders. The results of this test might explain why Donna miscarried and why she hadn't gotten pregnant with our embryos the first two rounds. It would also help us to determine which embryos to transfer this time. The drawbacks of the test are a five to ten percent error rate and a slight risk of damaging the embryo. Despite my loss of faith in statistical probability, I figured that collecting information that was ninety-percent accurate was better than obtaining no information at all.

On the appointed date, we returned to southern California for the egg retrieval and transfer. This time Dr. P. removed twenty-something eggs. Of them seventeen fertilized and were tested. Five days later we returned, with Donna, to his office to find out the results of the PGD and to transfer some embryos. Of the seventeen embryos a few had serious genetic problems like trisomy 18 and monosomy 21. The embryologist was unable to remove a cell or get a signal for another bunch of embryos. In the end it was determined that five of the embryos were normal. So we transferred those and hoped that our odds of having a viable pregnancy had improved. On the one hand I was happy that we had done PGD. We learned that some of our embryos were not viable and would probably not have implanted successfully or would have miscarried had they been transferred. But, on the other hand, it seemed unlikely that all or even most of the eighteen embryos we had transferred over the first three rounds of IVF were unviable. This test may have given us some information, but it was not definitive and it was still no guarantee of a successful pregnancy.

As the end of the tense two-week wait approached I knew that Donna wasn't pregnant. When I talked with her on the phone she avoided discussing pregnancy symptoms and seemed less bubbly than usual. My fears were confirmed by Dr. P.'s nurse and then Donna. Donna had in fact taken a home pregnancy test but was required by the agency to leave the dirty work to the nurse. At this point I was utterly demoralized and frustrated. If Dr. P. had bothered to call I'm sure he would have accused my poor old eggs of producing unviable embryos. But this time, we had fair proof that the embryos were likely to have been perfectly healthy. We still had no explanations and no incentive to keep trying or even to quit. Not knowing put us in a weird state of limbo. I had already decided that I wouldn't undergo any more rounds of IVF. I simply couldn't handle it physically or psychologically. We had a few frozen embryos from the earlier rounds of IVF, but there weren't too many and they weren't the best ones we'd produced. Roger and I now began a new debate: donor egg and a gestational surrogate or adoption.

## Chapter 7

While Donna was recovering from another D and C, Roger and I had endless debates about our next move. Despite little evidence and my lack of conviction that I was infertile, I was certain that I would not undergo any more rounds of IVF. By this time, I felt that I had experienced more than enough pointless bodily abuse, and I was done with it. Since Dr. P. wasn't volunteering advice about quitting or pursuing other avenues, I had to draw the line. The problem was that I was not enthusiastic about either of my alternatives; I was tepid about adoption and strongly opposed to using donor eggs.

I continued to research adoption options. Possibly, since I was already ambivalent about adopting and because Roger saw it as "a last resort," in my inquiries I looked for every possible flaw or horror story I could find. I focused on the tragic cases of children with fetal alcohol syndrome, drug addiction, and severe developmental problems from months or years of neglect and abuse in orphanages. Instead of concentrating on the many wonderful adoption stories I knew, I brooded over an article by Dan Savage, in *The New York Times*, about his experience with an open adoption of a child of a homeless, mentally unstable woman. Even though he seemed delighted with fatherhood and had no regrets about adopting, I was deeply disturbed by his story. The child did not have great genes, and his unreliable, mentally ill mother still made periodic appearances in his life. At the same time, I certainly knew that I or any healthy, conscientious, intelligent person could give birth to a severely impaired, sickly child, but it seemed to me that the odds of serious problems were greater when adopting than when controlling for, at least, some of the variables.

Given our experiences with my own pregnancies and IVF with a gestational surrogate, I was no believer in the miracles of science, or in my own genes, or in Donna's flawless uterus. In adoption's defense, it was pretty much a sure thing. There were plenty of babies out there who needed parents, and one way or another we would be able to adopt one. Surrogacy and IVF, on the other hand, were a gamble. We could spend hundreds of thousands of dollars, use the finest physicians in the country, have good odds, and still not get a child. There was no guarantee of success. However, with IVF and surrogacy one mostly hears the stories with happy endings. People don't talk about their failures in this domain. I suspect that many of the people who don't end up with children via IVF, adopt.

To me, resorting to an egg donor and a gestational surrogate was the final insult. After all that I had undergone, both physically and emotionally, I felt that my role as a mother and all that I had experienced were completely negated. I would neither carry a baby nor help produce one. Using a donor egg seemed almost tawdry and raised some complicated ethical issues. My husband would be creating a child with another woman. At least with adoption Roger and I would be on equal footing. We'd both be raising the child produced by another man and woman. But here, I had unsuccessfully given birth to two babies and then been through four rounds of IVF, and now my husband was effectively replacing me with a fertile twenty-something year old. I was also worried that if our egg donor had made previous donations or would make future ones, or had children of her own, our child would have unknown biological half siblings. While the odds of a future incestuous relationship developing between the half siblings were slim, I still wanted no part in creating such a potential scenario. Although I knew that I should tell our child that he or she came from a donor egg, I certainly didn't want to. I was haunted by the idea that many years from now, when our child was a huffy adolescent having an argument with me, he or she would lash out declaring that I was not his or her real mother. I couldn't bear that. Everything about this picture was much too close to science fiction for my taste. Finally, and perhaps most frustrating of all, even this was no sure thing. A young, healthy egg donor gave us better odds, but IVF with a surrogate was a complex process with many unknowns, and this too might fail.

Since Roger wasn't budging about adoption, I tried finding ways to rationalize using an egg donor. One of us had to compromise or we would never have a child. The question was whether I could not only live with but fully embrace something that I found deeply problematic. I reflected on a conversation with the woman who first talked to us at our initial consultation at the surrogacy agency. She had used a surrogate and an egg donor because, she explained, she wanted to give her husband a child, and she was unable to herself. At the time that struck me as the martyr-like comment of a 1950's housewife. However, upon reconsidering her statement, I wondered if she had committed a tremendously generous act for someone she loved. I wasn't so sure that I could be that generous or selfless, but it was worth thinking about.

I also had a long conversation with our counselor, Susan, from the surrogacy agency, who had used donor eggs but had carried her own babies. Talking to her was particularly helpful because she was frank and knew a great deal about surrogacy and egg donation both professionally and personally. Susan listened to and addressed many of my concerns and emphasized that I had to feel comfortable about using a donor egg. If I was ashamed or resentful of needing an egg donor, my discomfort would cause problems now and in the future. And that was precisely my main concern. How could I agree to something like this if I was only grudgingly acquiescing?

The surrogacy agency worked closely with an egg donation agency, so they smoothed the path for us a bit and connected us to their egg donor data base. This way we could at least look at some available egg donors, familiarize ourselves with the process, and get a sense of who was out there donating her eggs. My initial searches through the data base only discouraged me from agreeing to use an egg donor and fueled my concerns. Perhaps because the agency was based in southern California the donors who signed up were of a particular type that one might be less likely to find in New England. An astonishing number were blond or bottle blonds and had had breast implants. Many boasted of their breast sizes, which amazed me. Why would I care about a woman's boob size? I wasn't looking for a date. If she produced a male child for us, how would her breast size be relevant? Finally, plastic surgery gave us no inkling of what this woman really looked like. I can't say that I was particularly impressed by the talents, intelligence, or accomplishments of many of the egg donors. For the most part, they were merely pretty, young, and probably fertile. That wasn't good enough for me.

With Roger's assistance, we figured out how to narrow our search and view profiles of egg donors who had other claims to fame than possessing big breasts. Though I was still underwhelmed, we did manage to find a few egg donors who seemed intelligent, sane, healthy, interesting, and attractive. Selecting an egg donor forces one to pinpoint one's values. Evidently, many potential parents in southern California were hoping for daughters who looked like Barbie dolls. While we were not averse to having an attractive child, we weren't going to consider a Barbie unless she had a high IQ, a decent education, good health and family medical history, and seemed stable and interesting. Roger and I ended up finding a few potential egg donors who looked like they could be my relatives, though not twin sisters, appeared to be intelligent, healthy, creative, thoughtful, and kind. Obviously, there are limits to what can be determined from a few pages of a web site profile. I was somewhat reassured that there were good donors out there, but I was still apprehensive because none of them ultimately, was me.

After further discussion with Roger and Susan and friends, and more consideration, I finally agreed to engage an egg donor. We had already invested so much time, thought, energy, and money in surrogacy that using an egg donor seemed like a small step compared to adoption. By this point surrogacy was a known, even with an egg donor, whereas adoption felt like starting from scratch. Also, throughout my misadventures, I discovered that I could accept and do things I would have once rejected. So I got in touch with the egg donation company that was affiliated with our surrogacy agency. The style and nature of the egg donor agency differed dramatically from that of the surrogacy agency. Egg donation seems to be more overtly about money than surrogacy. Most of the egg donors admit to needing money to pay off debts or college loans and then mention wanting to help infertile women as an aside. Many are happy to be anonymous donors, don't want to meet or know much, if anything about the babies they help create, and see this, in part, as a good deed business transaction. For gestational surrogates, on the other hand, money is not the primary motivation, even though many of them could use the added income. The director of the egg donor agency reflected the culture of egg donation. She was efficient, a bit officious, and good at contacting and procuring egg donors. She maddeningly referred to the donors as "ladies," making them sound like call girls and praised, with great hyperbole, their various attributes. After reading our application and profile and talking to me, Lisa, the director, recommended specific donors whom she felt fit our specifications. Although she was trying to help us and expedite the process, she definitely did not get us. I was taken aback by her presumptuousness; it seemed to me that it is awfully difficult to choose an appropriate egg donor for someone else, especially someone you hardly know. Lisa kept recommending tall, attractive donors who were outrageously fertile. Besides that, they weren't very appealing to us. Susan suggested I ignore Lisa, and so I did. After further searching and fretting, we finally found a few donors we liked.

Lisa explained that we should identify three donors and rank them. She would contact them and let us know who was available. According to Lisa, all three donors turned out to be enthusiastic and interested in working with us but were available only with various constraints. One was in the middle of an egg donation cycle for another couple. She was happy to do it again for us in a couple of months. The other was in school full time, lived on the West Coast and would have to schedule a cycle around her school vacations. The third one lived on the East Coast and also was a full-time college student. She too had to plan the donation around her school schedule and factor in travel time. We decided to "reserve" the donor who was in the middle of a cycle for another couple. In a couple of weeks we could find out if she responded well to IVF and if so, engage her as our egg donor.

After a couple of weeks, Lisa called to let us know that our possible egg donor had a bad reaction to the hormones and had to terminate the cycle midway. While we were disappointed that this donor was no longer feasible and felt sorry for the other couple, we were relieved that we were spared the failed cycle. We now turned to our next choice of egg donor, Megan, who lived on the West Coast. Megan was a previous, successful egg donor, so we knew she was a good bet. Lisa contacted her and we made arrangements to begin IVF as soon as she was screened. The goal was to do the egg retrieval right after her final exams in December. Once again, we filled out tons of paperwork and signed contracts and checks. Although we never actually met Megan, our indirect dealings with her were utterly maddening. According to Susan, our counselor and the egg donation agency, she was irresponsible about forwarding records and returning phone calls. Everyone enjoyed talking with her when she was reachable, but she was hard to contact. I was livid. I felt like we were being toyed with, and I was in no mood for games. Finally, when deadlines were approaching and important paperwork was still missing, Susan basically gave Megan an ultimatum: either she fly to southern California for an interview with her and a complete psychological and medical screening or she was out. If there were any problems or concerns in any of the tests, Susan recommended that we drop Megan. After a long day for everyone involved, Susan called to let us know that Megan passed with flying colors. She charmed everyone, showed up on time, and seemed healthy, intelligent, energetic, artistic, and sensitive. And so we commenced round five.

Even though it was hard to accept that I would have no biological role in the creation of our child, I was relieved not to be undergoing another round of IVF. Dr. P.'s nurse kept us informed of Megan's progress throughout the cycle. Her hormone levels were good, and she was developing plenty of eggs, though far fewer than I had, I couldn't help noting. I spoke to Donna regularly as well, who as usual, was growing a nice uterine lining and had appropriate hormone levels. Just as I did, Megan flew down to Orange County a couple of days before the retrieval and was monitored at the clinic there. Before Megan's scheduled egg retrieval, Roger had to go to the clinic to make his sperm donation. We never met Megan, which was deliberate on both of our parts. As far as I was concerned, there already were too many people involved in our efforts to have a baby. I couldn't handle any more baby-related relationships. The natural way of making a baby simply involved two people in the privacy of their bedroom. I had accepted that this would not be so in our case. But, I didn't feel that I needed to involve the entire West Coast of the United States in forming our family. Megan returned home the day after the retrieval, and we returned to Orange County for the transfer three days later.

The day of the transfer set a new record for bad treatment and aggravation at Dr. P.'s office. Donna, Steve, Roger, and I arrived at Dr. P.'s clinic at 8:30 AM, for what we were told was his first appointment of the day. When we all checked in, the waiting room was empty but began to fill up soon after. We were kept waiting for over an hour and a half. When Donna asked when we could expect to be seen, she was told that Dr. P. had not arrived yet. Had he overslept, decided to go out to brunch or surfing with his family? We were finally called in to the exam room. Dr. P. made his grand appearance, offered no apology or explanation for his lateness, and proceeded as if everything was as it should be. He informed us that there were twelve embryos and all looked great. He seemed positively ecstatic about the quality of the embryos, and in turn the eggs, as if the fact that Megan was young and fertile were a special talent. In fact, since the embryos all appeared to be developing beautifully and were basically indistinguishable from one another, he suggested that we return in another two days for the transfer so that he could see if some were stronger than others. He said that waiting until day five would not improve the odds of a pregnancy, but he would transfer only two embryos on day five as opposed to three today. We were expected to give him an answer immediately. I was seething with anger. Why hadn't he warned us of this outcome? In previous cycles he had said that embryos prefer the womb to a Petri dish, so wasn't it then preferable to transfer them earlier rather than later? Did it occur to him that Roger and I had flown down there for the transfer and that Roger and Steve had already taken off countless time from work and Donna from caring for her own children? If he had shown the slightest bit of regard for us as human beings with responsibilities and lives outside the fertility clinic, I wouldn't have been half as angry. Roger asked if we could talk it over in another room and get back to him shortly.

Our two-minute long conversation cost us at least another half an hour of pointless waiting. While Roger and I were chatting, or I was throwing a fit in an adjacent exam room, Dr. P. went off to deal with another patient. When he returned, we informed him that we wanted to do the transfer that day. Our odds of a pregnancy were the same, and the chances of defective embryos from the eggs of a healthy twenty-five year old with great genes were pretty slim. Dr. P. nodded and praised Donna and her fabulous uterus. While I was pleased that he was complimentary to Donna, I found it insensitive of him to flatter everyone else involved in the process and treat me as if I was some disinterested party. I couldn't wait to be done with the fertility clinic. I was exhausted and disgusted with the entire process. The transfer took place and we returned to the hotel with Donna for the usual confinement period and wait.

By now, since Donna and I were practically old friends and certainly old pros at this, Donna decided to take a home pregnancy test a few days before her scheduled blood test and give me the news herself. Neither one of us found much reason to withhold or delay information. Much to everyone's delight, Donna was pregnant. We were all immensely relieved and figured that maybe Dr. P. had been correct after all. My eggs, abundant as they were, may not have been the best quality. After only one try Donna became pregnant with embryos formed from a young, vibrant donor. At this point, I also felt more confident that this pregnancy would actually last, since the embryo or embryos were probably healthy. Donna's hormone levels were good and suggested that she was likely to be carrying only one or at most twins. This was all very positive, encouraging news for us. Perhaps this might be the low-risk pregnancy we had all been waiting for.

Just as Donna was approaching week six of pregnancy, I flew down to Orange County for the ultrasound. I'm not going to say the first ultrasound, since by now I had had and seen countless sonograms that were either the bearers of misleading good tidings or the bearers of accurate bad tidings. I was apprehensive about returning to Dr. P.'s office and waiting those few seconds before he analyzed what he saw on the ultrasound. By this time, I had numerous negative associations with flying to Orange County, staying there, the waiting area in John Wayne Airport, and Dr. P.' s exam rooms. My flight to Orange County was delayed over an hour, which added to my anxieties. It turned out that Dr. P. outlated me anyway. Donna and I still sat in the waiting area for more than an hour before we were seen.

The ultrasound finally got underway, and Donna and I stared intently at the monitor, trying to decipher the gray, amorphous shapes. It looked to me like there were two blobs, one fluid and slightly elongated and the other a more typical looking embryo. Dr. P. at first couldn't tell how many embryos there were, and he appeared concerned. After a bit of probing and measuring, he concluded that there was only one, which didn't seem to have a heartbeat. However, Dr. P. wasn't certain about the heartbeat. He could see a lighter colored spot that may have been the beginnings of a heart. He also cautioned that it was very early in the pregnancy, and sometimes it was difficult to find a heartbeat this early. Perhaps the embryo got off to a slow start. Dr. P. wasn't optimistic, but he also wasn't hopeless. He gave the embryo a twenty percent chance of surviving and recommended that we return in a week for another ultrasound. By then he could get a better read. Donna started to cry, and I felt utterly deflated and in complete disbelief. I couldn't stand much more of this. Why couldn't we have a typical, roller coaster-free pregnancy? We had all of the ingredients of a low-risk pregnancy, and it still wasn't working. Yet again, the ultrasound provided nothing but an unexpected twist, an unpleasant surprise, and no remedy.

Donna and I went out to lunch and discussed our predicament. Oddly enough, we were both angry and frustrated more than sad. There was still no good explanation for this failed pregnancy other than bad luck. Approximately twenty percent of pregnancies end in miscarriages, and this, unfortunately may have been one of those. It didn't necessarily mean that there was something wrong with the embryos. One of Donna's favorite expressions is "Welcome to my world." Unfortunately, as far as pregnancy was concerned, she had entered my world.

After our venting session of a lunch, Donna returned home and I drove back to the airport completely distracted and self-absorbed. I was so busy brooding, that I almost side-swiped someone in my absurdly monstrous SUV that the rental car agency inflicted on me. I then sat around the increasingly-hateful John Wayne Airport waiting to board the plane and trying to reach Roger who was at a conference in Europe. Going to the ultrasound by myself was a big mistake. This was the second time that I was without Roger when finding out particularly bad news. When I finally reached him, our discussion was repeatedly interrupted by a poor connection, and I was completely frustrated with Roger, our cell phone service, Dr. P., ultrasounds, Orange County, and pretty much everything and everyone. I was stuck alone, frustrated and upset watching Disneyland-bound families dressed in Mickey Mouse attire getting off the inbound flight.

When I arrived home, I got in touch with Susan, our counselor, who was shocked and dismayed by our news. She volunteered to accompany Donna to the next ultrasound. She didn't see any reason for me to fly down to Orange County for more disappointment. If and when there was a positive, healthy pregnancy, I should see the sonogram but not before. Even though I wanted to be involved in as much of the pregnancy as I was able to, I was immensely relieved to avoid Dr. P.'s office, the site of bad news. By this point I felt as if I might have to move to another part of the country. My neighborhood was tainted with bad associations, and now so was southern California.

The next week Donna returned for another ultrasound accompanied by Susan. I spent the morning with my cell phone in one hand and the house phone in the other. Finally, Susan and Donna called with surprising news. The embryo had a heartbeat! It wasn't as strong as it should have been, but it was there, and the embryo seemed to be growing properly. Dr. P. now gave us an eighty percent chance of a successful outcome. I was cautiously happy. It was still very early in the pregnancy, and the embryo was clearly getting off to a shaky start. Dr. P. wanted to see Donna in another week for an ultrasound. Susan said that she would join Donna at Dr. P.'s office. If things looked good by week ten, then I would fly to Orange County to see our developing baby.

On the day of the ultrasound for week eight, I waited by the phone again. This time Dr. P.'s assistant called saying that Dr. P. was on the line and wanted to talk to me. This could only be bad news. Dr. P. called, unprompted, only once before about the quadruplet pregnancy fiasco. Dr. P. explained that the embryo no longer had a heartbeat and was not growing. He recommended that Donna have another D and C so that he could test the tissue to determine if the embryo had any genetic disorders. He also wanted to do an antibody test on Donna to see if she was developing antibodies that were causing her body to reject our embryos. Finally, he suggested that Roger be tested for Y chromosome abnormalities. When I had asked Dr. P., on more than one occasion, if there might be a problem with Donna or Roger, I was dismissed as if I had asked an idiotic question. Clearly, it had to be my defective eggs that were at fault. Now he wanted to test Donna and Roger?! Why hadn't he tested them earlier, say after the second failed transfer? It was nice to know that I finally was not to blame. Perhaps my eggs weren't so bad after all. This was small comfort, however. It was now possible that we may not have had to use an egg donor after all. Because of Dr. P.'s failure to listen or examine every angle, we were out many more thousands of dollars, had wasted numerous months of people's lives, and experienced egregious disappointment and loss. It was nice that Dr. P. was trying to find an explanation, but couldn't he have ordered these tests about a year earlier?

About a week or two after all of the tests were conducted and cultured, Dr. P.'s nurse called. The embryonic tissue that was retrieved from the D and C was normal. Roger had no chromosomal abnormalities, and Donna was not producing antibodies that were causing her to reject our embryos. However, Donna was also given a glucose test, which indicated that she is hypoglycemic. Dr. P.'s nurse explained that a recent study showed that abnormal glucose levels can affect the ability to get pregnant or maintain a pregnancy especially when using IVF. The nurse said that Donna would be put on Metformin, a drug in the insulin family, and that we could then proceed with another cycle. Although Dr. P. wasn't certain that Donna's glucose levels were the cause of our repeated failures, he thought that Metformin might help and that this problem should be addressed. When I asked the nurse further questions about Metformin and the implications of taking this drug, she was unable to answer me. It seems to me that Dr. P., a reproductive endocrinologist should have been on the phone. It also appeared that he was making quite a few assumptions without conferring with us or informing us first. Perhaps if Donna were better informed she might not have agreed to take Metformin. If Roger and I had been given more information, we might have decided that the risks were too high for Donna and a pregnancy.

I called Susan as soon as I received this "information." She knew nothing about this prognosis but said that she would investigate the matter. She also recommended that I call or email Dr. P. with a list of questions and concerns. I opted for email since I figured I would have to wait at least a week to schedule a phone call. In the meantime I spoke to a scientist friend and Dr. M., and Roger talked to his internist about our situation. All raised concerns about Donna's increased risk for gestational diabetes and all recommended that we stop working with her. She was too high a risk. Why hadn't Dr. P. offered such advice or warned of such risks?

In my first email to Dr. P. I wrote: "I have a few questions about Donna's glucose levels and the treatment she'll be starting. Do you think that her low glucose level affected her ability to become pregnant or stay pregnant in the last five rounds of IVF? Why is she being treated with Metformin if she's not diabetic?" He replied: "Her glucose levels reflect an over production of insulin in response to glucose and other carbohydrates. She is insulin resistant and therefore over-produces insulin. Her over-production of insulin is likely a combination of an inherent defect that she has that has been exacerbated by her weight. These elevated insulin levels may contribute to early pregnancy loss and reproductive failure. The data on this subject are still very preliminary but metformin is a Class B drug and it is worth trying in Donna's situation." He answered my medical questions but did not consider the implications of continuing to work with a surrogate who was over-producing insulin and was obese.

So, I wrote him another note in which I asked: "Just how concerned should we be about Donna's ability to become pregnant and maintain a pregnancy? Does this mean that she is also at higher risk for gestational diabetes? Is the Metformin likely to take care of her glucose/insulin issues? Why was she able to get pregnant naturally with her own children and carry her four children to term with no problems?" Dr. P. wrote back:

"Yes, she is as higher risk for developing gestational diabetes, although the incidence is significantly reduced if she continues to take the metformin during her gestation. The fact that she did not previously have gestational diabetes is also a good sign. She was younger and probably thinner when she got pregnant on her own. Increasing age and weight both increase insulin resistance and so it might be a problem now whereby it wasn't a problem previously." He finally acknowledged that Donna was at risk for gestational diabetes but still said nothing about whether it was a good idea to continue with Donna. Wasn't the point of using a surrogate to have a low-risk pregnancy? I could do a high-risk pregnancy all by myself.

Still frustrated with Dr. P.'s insistence on addressing one problem while failing to see the big picture, I wrote: "Roger and I are quite concerned about Donna working out as a surrogate. If you were screening her to be a surrogate and had all the information you have on her today, would you recommend her?" He simply responded, "no". Well there was our answer. Couldn't he have called and told us this after receiving the results of her glucose test and saved everyone time, money, and aggravation? Although a glucose test is not part of the standard screening for surrogates, given that Donna was overweight and that she was being screened for numerous other things, couldn't he have tested her earlier instead of dragging out this nightmare for a year and a half? Would Dr. P. have simply let us continue, failed cycle after failed cycle, indefinitely? Was he at all concerned about Donna's health and Roger and I having a viable, full-term baby? Did he remember why we came to him in the first place? I was furious. I didn't really want to sue Dr. P. He hadn't exactly conducted malpractice. I wanted my money back and an apology—two things I was well aware I would never receive. I knew that there were no guarantees in the fertility business, but I did expect the doctor to have our best interests in mind and to be forthcoming. I felt like we'd been had.

After discussing our predicament with Roger and forwarding the email exchanges with Dr. P. to Susan, I called Susan. We all agreed that it would be wise to stop working with Donna and find a new surrogate. Susan assured me that we would receive first priority and be matched with a new surrogate as soon as possible. I certainly didn't want to drop Donna. She had been tremendously generous and kind to us. She was cheerful, conscientious, and easy to deal with. She had wasted a year and a half of her life and burdened her own family for pretty much nothing. Her intention was to help us, and now, it turned out that she might be the source of the problem. Susan and I decided that it would be best if I called Donna and broke the news to her, and then Susan would follow up. I felt like I was breaking up with a boyfriend.

Breaking up with Donna was sad but went better than I anticipated. As always, she was understanding and gracious. She grasped our reasons and that our goal was to have a child. If she couldn't provide one for us, then someone else would have to. We've talked many times since we ended our official surrogate relationship and continue to remain friends. I wasn't particularly excited about starting over with a new surrogate and developing this weirdly intimate relationship with another stranger. I figured that Donna turned out to be a very pleasant surprise. I was more comfortable with our partnership than I would ever have imagined. Perhaps, in the future, our next adventure with a gestational surrogate and in baby making might work out on both fronts.

## Chapter 8

There is no instant gratification when it comes to making babies the new-fangled way. At least the old-fashioned process involves pleasure. Waiting to get re-matched with another gestational carrier required a good deal of patience, phone calls, emails, and paperwork and produced tremendous anxiety. In reality, we didn't even have to wait very long, but it didn't feel that way since we had been doing nothing but waiting for years; every extra day or week felt like many months and brought new worries. After a few angst-ridden weeks we received the profile of a surrogate who had already read our file and expressed interest in working with us. The new gestational surrogate, Celia, and her husband, Miguel, live near Los Angeles and have two school-aged children of their own. A few years earlier Celia carried twins to term for another couple and had become pregnant on the first try. She had a great track record. In her letter, she seemed upbeat and pleasant. We were also assigned a new counselor by the surrogacy agency since Celia lives in a different area from Donna. I had found our previous counselor, Susan, to be helpful, supportive, responsible, and wise and was disappointed to lose her as an advisor. Our new counselor, Marsha, wasn't as warm or easy to talk to as Susan, but had good credentials and was very experienced. Marsha suggested that I call Celia, and if we liked each other, she would help arrange a meeting in Los Angeles.

My phone conversation with Celia went surprisingly smoothly. She was easy to talk to, warm, and seemed to have common sense. So after a series of exchanges with all parties involved, we set up a meeting in Los Angeles with Marsha, Celia, Miguel, Roger, and me. Marsha also recommended that I change fertility physicians since I was not happy with my experience at Dr. P.'s clinic and particularly frustrated with him. Despite the tedious logistics involved in switching doctors, I was relieved to be done with Dr. P.'s office and Orange County and all of their negative associations. Changing the variables, I hoped, would have its merits.

About two weeks after receiving Celia's profile, Roger and I flew down to L.A. to meet her and her husband. Since Marsha wanted to meet us herself and introduce us to Celia, we arranged to talk with her first at the surrogacy agency where Celia and Miguel would join us later. It was strange to return to the surrogacy agency after two and a half years. It seemed comfortable and familiar even though we had only been there once. Perhaps because we had been in contact with so many employees of the agency over the years, we didn't feel like strangers. What was odd was meeting Marsha and feeling like we were being assessed again. Although she was probably just trying to get to know us and was looking out for Celia, I felt annoyed by her repeated questions and judgments. We had already been interviewed and had more than proven ourselves as responsible, decent people who treated their surrogate well. She asked us repeatedly if we got along with Donna even though we responded with an enthusiastic "yes" each time. I had to restrain myself from sarcastically saying, "Why don't you call Susan or Donna who will give you the lowdown on us." By this point Roger and I had more than shown our commitment to being parents and to the entire surrogacy process. We didn't need a new round of interrogation.

Although I understand the legal and practical reasons why, it is unfair and irksome that there are no standards or regulations to becoming parents for people who can have children naturally, while there are endless tests to pass for parents who adopt or use a surrogate. In the realm of parenting, biology is privileged. If you have sex and get pregnant, then you are qualified to be a parent. Drug addicts, alcoholics, pedophiles, and abusers can procreate. In adoption and surrogacy there are numerous hoops to jump through including psychological, medical, legal, and financial criteria. The time, energy, stamina, and numerous qualifications involved in adopting a child or having one through a surrogate or through IVF are better measures of someone's capability, commitment and desire to have a child than an accidental conception after someone forgets to use contraception. Roger and I had been tried and tested and just wanted Marsha to take care of logistical issues and introduce us to Celia. We could handle the rest.

After a prolonged conversation with Marsha, Celia and Miguel finally arrived, much to Roger's and my relief. Marsha made the introductions, took care of her business with us, and left us to go out to dinner and get to know each other. Dinner with Celia and Miguel was delightful. There was no awkwardness and making conversation was easy. We chatted about work, family, schools, hobbies, and of course, surrogacy and pregnancy. Neither Roger nor I was particularly worried about Celia. Maybe because we had already had a positive relationship with Donna and were familiar with the various aspects of surrogacy, we were more open to accepting a surrogate and much less suspicious and nervous. Perhaps we should have been more critical and were too eager to get started again and too trusting in the surrogacy agency's screening powers. Apparently Celia felt the same way. When we returned home, Marsha called to let us know that we were "officially" matched with Celia and that we should arrange for contracts to be drawn up and doctor's appointments.

*The Maternity Labyrinth*

I had actually already scheduled an appointment with the fertility doctor that Marsha recommended and whom Celia had already worked with in her first surrogacy. The consultation was set a few days later in Los Angeles. Once again I flew to L.A. for a meeting with Dr. R. whom Marsha described as "highly ethical and kind." That alone sounded like an improvement over my last fertility center experience. In addition to being a *mensch*, Dr. R. was a highly respected reproductive endocrinologist, professor at a medical school, and author who specialized in infertility in older women. Though I still wasn't convinced that I was infertile and was not thrilled about being in the older woman category, I could admit that he seemed like an appropriate doctor for me.

The prospect of seeing a new doctor and renewing the baby-making process with a new surrogate revived some dilemmas about using my own eggs versus our frozen embryos created with the donor eggs. If Donna may have been the source or part of the problem then perhaps I should try IVF again but with a different surrogate. As I considered the process again, I literally felt queasy. I couldn't imagine volunteering to experience the frightening moods and horrible headaches another time. Also, even if I was relatively fertile, my eggs were still not likely to be the greatest quality. Many were likely to have chromosomal abnormalities which would lead to miscarriages or no pregnancy at all. The odds of a pregnancy using my almost forty-two year old eggs were pretty poor. We had a couple of frozen embryos from one of my previous rounds of IVF, but they weren't the best quality. It seemed that our strongest chances for having a healthy baby would entail using the frozen embryos of the egg donor. I was willing to engage in a discussion with Dr. R. about this and possibly entertain trying another round of IVF. Having a child in the near future rather than prolonging this process was more important to me at this point.

From the moment I entered Dr. R.'s office, which is located in a high rise near a medical center, I noticed a vast difference in the ambiance from that of Dr. P.'s office. I was greeted warmly by the receptionists who knew my name and were awaiting my arrival. Instead of ignoring me or treating me as if I were intruding, they chatted with me and kept me posted about when the doctor would be available. Like every other fertility clinic and obstetrician's office I had frequented, the walls of this office were decorated with bulletin boards covered with photos of babies. I suppose it was meant to instill confidence and hope in new patients and even serve as a source of inspiration to them. At times I felt a twinge of jealousy looking at the pictures of all the cute, smiling infants. I also must confess that I desperately wanted to have our baby's photo displayed on one of those boards. I fantasized about sending birth announcements and photos to our numerous doctors. Shortly after I arrived and in the middle of my usual baby announcement-sending reverie, Dr. R. came out to the waiting area to greet me and usher me into his office. I spent close to an hour and a half talking with Dr. R. He listened carefully, was attentive, took notes, and presented his opinions and recommendations. I was relieved to learn that there were fertility doctors who were both smart and competent, as well as sensitive and kind.

Dr. R.'s analysis of my situation didn't differ radically from Dr. P.'s. He was clear and blunt about the probability of getting pregnant at my age. However, instead of referring to my age as if it were an accusation or simply calling me older, he gave me the facts and told me encouraging stories. I guess he figured that I knew the discouraging tales first hand. Based on the information I gave him, Dr. R. believed that Donna was probably okay and not the source of our failed pregnancies and miscarriages. He also did not think that I am infertile nor needed an egg donor. Basically, he thought that we had had a lot of bad luck. According to him, our "success rate," that is the quadruplet pregnancy, was quite good, given the total number of embryos implanted. In order to achieve a pregnancy after age forty, one needed "persistence and gentleness." He was not an advocate of PGD or other invasive procedures, like assisted hatching, since embryos created from older eggs are weaker and tend to be damaged by too much manipulation. He presented a variety of possibilities, including trying to get pregnant myself and going on full bed rest in a hospital, and left it to me to decide what to do.

Attempting pregnancy again, which would entail bed rest and a cerclage and a six month hospital stay, was completely out of the question. Just because there were anecdotes of successful pregnancies under those conditions did not mean it would work for me. In fact it hadn't worked for me, and there was no reason to think that it would a second time. I had also long ago come to terms with using a surrogate. Why would I put myself, a pregnancy, and a baby at risk if I had a healthier, safer alternative? Using my own eggs with a gestational carrier seemed slightly more reasonable to me but when presented with the odds, I was discouraged. There was a six percent chance of implantation per embryo with eggs of a woman my age. Dr. R. thought that I was likely to get pregnant with repeated attempts. I had already tried four times. If he could have guaranteed that we would have a viable pregnancy after one more round of IVF, I would have done it. But he couldn't. I was all for persistence. As a matter of fact, I felt that I deserved an award for persistence. One friend told me that I'd had the longest gestation of anyone she'd known. I just couldn't stand another round of IVF, particularly when the odds of success weren't very good. Our young, hearty frozen embryos and our hale, proven surrogate seemed to be a much better formula for success.

Because Roger and I and Celia were experienced with the legal and medical aspects of IVF and surrogacy and we would be using frozen embryos, I assumed that the process could begin in a mere matter of weeks. After all, there were no cycles to coordinate, Celia and I had already undergone medical screening, and we were all on board and eager to begin the process. Instead, it took over two months from the time we first met Celia and Miguel to the day she began to take hormones. The lawyers took their time drawing up contracts; Dr. R. wanted to do a mock transfer on Celia which had to coincide with her period that wouldn't arrive for another three weeks after my consultation with him. If all looked good, we would have to wait until the following month to begin Celia's drug regimen.

In the mean time I arranged to have our embryos transported from the Orange County facility to the Los Angeles office. I was told, repeatedly, by everyone involved that it would be simple to move the embryos. They did it all the time; they even shipped them from over seas. Moving them from one part of southern California to another, I was told, was a joke. It turned out to be a very bad joke and major nuisance that involved too many parties, none of whom would take any responsibility for managing the process. Basically, the L.A. center asked me to arrange with another lab to provide a dry shipper to be delivered to the Orange County clinic, which would then fill the container with the embryos and have them sent by Fed Ex to Los Angeles. The container arrived in Orange County a day later than scheduled, and the O.C. lab in turn filled and shipped the container the next day without informing me or the Los Angeles office. After days of many frantic phone calls in which I tried to locate the embryos, and was given conflicting answers by everyone I talked to, I learned that the embryos were simply sent out later than initially planned and were safe and sound. I was also relieved to learn that instead of being sent to Tennessee, as Fed Ex typically routes all of its packages, they were shipped straight to L.A. Fed Ex's tracking system was the only easy and efficient part of the whole process. I'm convinced that it would have been easier to transport the embryos myself. Miraculously, they arrived, seemingly intact, to Dr. R.'s lab.

By this point, I was becoming discouraged once again. Nothing was running as smoothly or quickly as I had hoped. Dr. R.'s nurse was rather non-committal about when Celia would begin taking medications and Dr. R. was away on vacation. Then, just as I was approaching new heights of exasperation, Celia called to inform me that she got her period and just had an appointment with another doctor in Dr. R.'s practice, who started her on the drug protocol. In a little over two weeks, if she responded well to the drugs, Celia would be ready for the embryo transfer. I was stunned. Within twenty-four hours we went from having no plan to book your flights to L.A. because there may be a pregnancy in a few weeks.

However, lest Roger and I actually experience a moment of hope or relief, in my following conversation with Celia, after casually asking, Celia blithely informed me that she was not taking prenatal vitamins since she wasn't pregnant yet. I found it rather strange that she hadn't been taking them as soon as she started seeing Dr. R. The surrogacy agency explained to us, long ago, that surrogates were required to take prenatal vitamins as soon as they were under contract. Celia's obliviousness and the carelessness of Dr. R.'s nurse alarmed me. Celia also didn't seem to understand what bed rest entailed. Although fertility doctors prescribe varying degrees of bed rest after an embryo transfer, most recommend at least a day of relaxation. Celia believed that that included cleaning her house and running errands. It seems to me that even the most lenient form of bed rest would not entail scrubbing a kitchen floor and carrying sacks of groceries. Celia's cavalier attitude was worrying me. No doubt, she felt invulnerable to pregnancy problems and had complete faith in her powers of conception. Nonetheless, she would be carrying our baby and was presumably doing this to help a couple who had experienced numerous disappointments. Couldn't she at least feign concern and humor us, if nothing else?

By calling Marsha and Dr. R.'s nurse, I saw to it that Celia understood the requirements and limitations of bed rest and began taking prenatal vitamins. My concerns about Celia were also alleviated once I saw her again in Los Angeles. The fact of the matter was that I simply didn't know her very well and had to rely on a first impression and a few short phone calls to feel comfortable with her and trust her. Roger and I flew down to L.A. the night before the embryo transfer. The next morning we picked up Celia and took her to Dr. R.'s office for the procedure. In contrast to our experience at Dr. P.'s office, we weren't kept waiting for hours or ignored. The transfer went as smoothly as one can possibly go. Dr. R. informed us that the embryos defrosted perfectly and looked as good as fresh ones. He also praised Celia's uterus and cervix. This time, Roger and I were allowed to watch the procedure; Dr. R. transferred three embryos. Via the ultrasound monitor we could see the little white dots moving through the catheter into Celia's uterus. After Celia rested for a while, we took her home and spent the rest of the day with her. Our visit with Celia and her family was pleasant. By the end of the day we felt more confident in her and even cautiously hopeful.

However, by this point, it was no longer possible for me to be truly optimistic. Our odds of a pregnancy were about fifty percent, which is great in the world of IVF. But that still meant that there was a fifty percent chance of not having a pregnancy. We had to wait ten days to find out---ten frustrating days during which I could do nothing to expedite the process or influence the outcome. It was hard to refrain from interrogating Celia about how she was feeling even though I knew it was too early for her to experience signs of pregnancy and had been told by her that she never felt moody or sick when first pregnant. Throughout the years of dealing with pregnancy losses, IVF, and surrogacy I had gotten used to and quite adept at organizing and arranging appointments and medical and legal business. It seemed that I spend inordinate amounts of time calling, emailing, reading and signing documents, and traveling to Southern California. For those ten days I had nothing to arrange and was unable to control or affect the result we were hoping for.

Roger and I spent the day of Celia's blood test waiting for the phone to ring. After hearing nothing by noon I was becoming tense and at two o'clock, positively frantic. I called Celia, who hadn't heard from the clinic either. At three, Roger and I, cell phones in hand, decided to leave the house. I was in despair and had concluded that the nurse saved the bad news for the end of the day. Finally, at four thirty, my cell phone rang. It was Dr. R. himself, who informed us that Celia was pregnant! I had worked myself up into such a state, that it was hard to believe the good news. A few days later Celia went in for another blood test which indicated that her HcG levels were increasing appropriately. She was still pregnant. Despite knowing about our numerous misconceptions, many of our friends and family still didn't understand why we weren't elated about the pregnancy. I was incapable of having complete faith in the pregnancy, particularly this early and especially before the first ultrasounds. We had already seen a number of disappointing ultrasounds and experienced failed pregnancies despite positive Beta tests and solid HcG levels. Perhaps, if all was well by the end of the first trimester, I would feel unmitigated joy and excitement, though more likely, only when a healthy baby was born.

A few days after Celia's blood tests, Marsha called us to touch base and congratulate us on our happy news. Then, in her interrogatory manner, she asked how often I spoke to Celia and implied that Roger and I weren't spending enough time with her. I called Celia at least twice a week, just to chat, and more often to discuss doctor's appointments and procedures.

Roger and I were with her for the embryo transfer and planned to attend the ultrasounds and doctor's appointments. Did Celia or Marsha assume that Roger would take a leave from his job and then expect us to move to L.A. or rent a pied-a-terre there? Marsha noted that Celia told her that she hoped to see more of us now that she was pregnant; Marsha then mentioned that the other woman for whom Celia carried a baby, spent lots of time with her. That other couple also happened to live thirty minutes away from Celia and, as Marsha herself, inappropriately disclosed, the woman was nervous and micromanaged the whole pregnancy. Although, to some degree, Marsha was Celia's advocate, she should have been more sensitive to us and paid more attention to what we had undergone. After all, we were the ones who had been through multiple, consecutive losses and spent enormous sums of time and money on all of these procedures and trips to Southern California. Marsha also should have had the sense and tact to avoid comparing us to the other couple and to prevent Celia from doing so. We had every intention of treating Celia with kindness and respect and participating in the pregnancy as much as was reasonable and practical. We treated Celia much as we had Donna and had been praised by Susan for going above and beyond the call of duty. I wasn't convinced that Marsha interpreted Celia's comment correctly, and if she had, she should have intervened more thoughtfully and discussed reasonable expectations with both of us. I did not deserve to be chastised.

The appointment for the first ultrasound finally arrived. Roger and I flew to L.A. the evening before and met Celia at Dr. R.'s office. While she appeared to be in good spirits and was feeling well, I was a nervous wreck, had little appetite, and felt queasy. The kind, thoughtful treatment at Dr. R.'s office helped to calm me a bit. The first thing I noticed on the ultrasound monitor was two dark blobs, one with a tiny white speck and the other nothing. I immediately assumed that we had one viable embryo with a heartbeat and one without. After a good bit of prodding of Celia and measuring of the embryo sacs the doctor confirmed that there were three sacs but only one was growing properly and contained an embryo with a heartbeat. Dr. R. said that it was highly improbable that the other embryos were viable, but he would check again next week because there was a slight chance that one could be a late bloomer. Despite, what seemed to me, a problematic situation, Dr. R. seemed pleased. Apparently, this was not a repeat of any of our bad-news ultrasounds of the past. According to Dr. R., the empty sacs would not affect the healthy embryo and would eventually be absorbed rather than expelled or miscarried by Celia. A singleton pregnancy was safer than a twin pregnancy, and so as far as Dr. R. was concerned, this was a very positive finding. As of six weeks and three days, the pregnancy was progressing nicely. We then scheduled another ultrasound for the following week and went out to lunch with Celia.

One might expect me to experience enormous relief and begin to feel more optimistic about the pregnancy. However, I didn't. First, Celia was only six weeks pregnant, which was very early. Anything could happen at this point. Second, I wanted a clear cut, completely unambiguous ultrasound report. Why couldn't there be one or two normally developing embryos rather than one and a maybe. That second sac made me nervous. What if it turned out to have a heartbeat at week seven and then none at week eight as we had seen in our fifth round of IVF with Donna? I worried that I simply could no longer feel joy or trust in the entire pregnancy experience. Roger and Celia and Dr. R. seemed happy and worry free. Celia, so certain that nothing could go wrong, was even planning to go on a family vacation in a few weeks. But I couldn't help thinking about our previous disappointing ultrasounds and failed pregnancies. I still couldn't believe.

The week seven ultrasound confirmed that we still had one healthy embryo and supported that the other two black blots on the monitor were empty sacs. When I asked the doctor if it was safe to assume that Celia would not be carrying twins, she (another physician in the practice) responded, "Probably. But I've seen weirder things happen in this business." So a Lazarus-like embryo could rise after all. I longed for the time in this pregnancy when at least the doctors could view it as normal, low-risk, or typical.

The next ultrasound, one week later, also brought good news. Our embryo had a strong heartbeat and was still developing appropriately. The two other empty sacs remained just that, as Dr. R. had hoped and predicted. Things were beginning to look up. Roger and I then went out to lunch with Celia who told us that she and her family were planning (I use that term very loosely) an RV trip to San Francisco at the end of the week. From what I could discern, she hadn't looked at a map or guide book or made any reservations at RV parks. I believe that she was simply hoping to get into the RV and drive more or less northward. When Roger and I explained that it was impractical to drive an RV around San Francisco and impossible to park it, she seemed nonplused and didn't really understand our advice or warnings. Celia's easygoing, calm manner was pleasant and in a certain way, a nice counterpart to my, at this point, high-strung personality. But, at times, her laissez-faire, clueless mien worried me. I feared that despite having been pregnant three times, Celia remembered little about the dos and don'ts of pregnancy. She mentioned that she drank no liquids after 6:00

PM so that she wouldn't have to get up in the middle of the night to use the bathroom. Wasn't she aware that she was supposed to drink a lot of water to make sure that she was well hydrated while pregnant? She also told us that part of the interior of her house was being painted. When I suggested that she spend more time outdoors during the painting process, she looked at me as if I were mad. Her lack of awareness about basic common sense pregnancy behaviors made me wonder what else she was and wasn't doing that could potentially harm the fetus. From my perspective, she needed a refresher course: Pregnancy 101, but she assumed that all would be well since she had done this before seamlessly. I was utterly frustrated and furious. Why couldn't I, who followed every pregnancy rule to the letter of the law, carry a baby successfully, while Celia, who was uninformed and casual about everything, had carried multiple healthy babies to term.

Celia and her family ended up renting an RV and driving up to San Francisco during week nine of the pregnancy. Although it was probably perfectly safe to travel at that point, I was concerned that Celia hadn't checked with Dr. R. before planning her trip. Her leisurely style of travel did nothing to instill confidence in me about her level of common sense or responsibility. As of the day of her departure from the Los Angeles area, Celia had made no reservations at any RV parks, particularly near San Francisco and had hardly looked at a map or planned a route. Roger and I had offered to lend her our car to drive around San Francisco and invited her and her family to dinner, but Celia never really responded to either offer. She then called me while packing up the RV to ask if she could leave her dog at our house while visiting Alcatraz even though she knew that Roger is allergic to dogs. She also asked me to find some RV parks she could call. Despite my frustration with her, I located a number of parks and gave her the information. I heard nothing from her until two days later when she phoned early in the morning announcing that she was about ten minutes away from my house. She still had no where to park the RV in the Bay Area and had no plans. By that point I was done with playing travel agent. I gave her more phone numbers to call and figured I'd talk to her later that day. I still wasn't sure if I'd be cooking dinner for a large group that evening. That morning was the last time I heard from her until I finally reached her at home four days later after leaving multiple unreturned messages. As always, she was calm and said that she had finally found a place to stay near San Francisco and had enjoyed their trip. She seemed utterly oblivious about that fact that she had inconvenienced me and left me waiting for days wondering about her whereabouts and whether she'd be appearing at our doorstep for dinner or a place to stay. I didn't really care whether we had her family over for dinner or even saw her. In fact, I was just as happy to mind my own business and have her enjoy her family vacation. But I was thoroughly exasperated by her basic lack of manners and responsibility. I felt that I simply couldn't trust her to exercise good judgment. Things that I assumed were common sense, clearly weren't to everyone. I was coming to the conclusion that her three previous successful pregnancies were the results of dumb luck and not much else. And sure enough, the week ten ultrasound showed that everything was fine with our embryo. It didn't seem to matter what Celia did or didn't do. She had a fabulous uterus and luck was on her side.

I had assumed since it had been several months since Donna had had any surrogacy-related medical procedures and we were no longer under contract with her or involved with Dr. P. and his center that we would no longer have any financial dealings with the Orange County facility. But about a month or two after Donna's last visit to Dr. P. we received a substantial bill, despite having paid for all medical services before or at the time of the procedures. After many phone calls, it turned out that we had a significant credit. Apparently, the Orange County center took a $1,200.00 security deposit from us and would return it only after all fees, including lab charges which were processed slowly, were paid. We were told to call back in a month to determine how much credit we had left. This calling and deferring dance went on for some time. After about four months and numerous phone calls we received a refund for about $600.00 and were told that there might still be outstanding lab charges and we should check back in another month to determine if we had a remaining credit. Three months later I called and was again told that they were still reviewing our records. Finally after two weeks of persistent phone calls, I was told that we would be refunded another $900.00. If I hadn't caught the mistake and called repeatedly, would the fertility center simply have pocketed our $1,500.00? Neither Roger nor I even recalled that we had ever been informed that the O.C. center would hold our money as a security. Even if we were to give them the benefit of the doubt that they had explained their security deposit policy to us, they had a legal and ethical responsibility to return our money in a timely manner, perhaps even with interest, which they had probably been earning on our money. We had already shelled out a fortune to them for procedures that didn't work. Was it really necessary for them to steal our money and profit illegally from our losses?

In the middle of the twelfth week of the pregnancy, Roger flew to L.A. for the nuchal translucency test, a high level ultrasound in which the nuchal folds at the back of the developing baby's neck are measured to help determine the odds of Down syndrome and other chromosomal abnormalities. Unlike amniocentesis or CVS, the nuchal test is not definitive. Instead, the doctor calculates the statistical probability of the baby's chance of having a chromosomal abnormality based on the nuchal fold measurement, the mother's age, and the baby's gestational age. Despite having a very flexible schedule, I was unable to attend the procedure because Celia's appointment was scheduled, despite my pleading with the nurse, on my second day at a new job. Even though I wanted to see the ultrasound, I was also relieved to avoid another trip to Los Angles and felt that Roger needed to continue to share a greater part of the responsibility in dealing with Celia and the pregnancy than he had done with Donna. According to Roger, the ultrasound showed that the baby was healthy and growing properly. Two days later, the nurse called to report that our results were great and that there was only a one in ten thousand chance that our baby would have Down's or Trisomy 18. Further blood tests and the level two ultrasound performed at about the twentieth week would provide us with more information. Our twelve and a half week old pregnancy was progressing beautifully.

We saw Dr. R. for the last time at week thirteen of the pregnancy. If Celia's progesterone levels were appropriate, she would be taken off the hormone medications and "graduate" from the fertility doctor to her own obstetrician. Celia passed with honors and she was approved to see her own doctor. So we said our farewells and thank yous to Dr. R. and his staff and posted our baby's due date on the calendar of expected birth dates of baby's conceived in Dr. R.'s office. We left Dr. R.'s office with a far better attitude than we had when we parted ways with Dr. P. not only because we were expecting a baby and had successfully passed through the first trimester, but because we had been treated with kindness and sensitivity. Many friends counseled that I would forget the bitterness, anxiety, and disappointment I felt while I was being treated by Dr. P. I can't say that I forgot, but I certainly was less cynical about some fertility doctors and felt more hopeful about pregnancy and having a child in the near future.

## Chapter 9

Because we had successfully graduated from trimester one, we would no longer have weekly doctor appointments and ultrasounds. From week thirteen on, unless a problem arose, this pregnancy was deemed normal and low risk, which meant monthly appointments with Celia's obstetrician and only standard ultrasounds and tests. While I was enormously relieved to have passed through the most tenuous part of the pregnancy and to resume some semblance of my routine at home and work, no longer having to travel to Los Angeles every week, I feared ceding my illusion of control over the pregnancy. Since I was visiting Celia less frequently, I had fewer opportunities to see how the baby was developing, receive feedback and reassurance from doctors that all was well, and keep tabs on her. Instead, I had to rely on phone conversations in which Celia basically said that she felt fine and was hardly showing or experiencing any pregnancy symptoms. This was of little comfort to me, who had never experienced a regular pregnancy and could only see pregnancy as pathology.

To add to my feeling excluded from the pregnancy, Celia made it clear that she didn't want me to accompany her to her first appointment, at week thirteen, with her obstetrician, Dr. K. Even though I explained that I had no interest in observing him perform a gynecological exam on her but just wanted to meet him and ask him some questions, she insisted that she preferred to go alone. I could meet him at her next check up, during week seventeen. When I told Marsha of my concerns and interest in knowing Celia's doctor, she reassured me that Dr. K. was probably perfectly competent and that it was quite common for surrogates to see their obstetricians without the intended parents. She also warned me not to expect Dr. K. to treat me as the patient or even the mother of the developing baby. From his perspective, Celia was his patient, and I had nothing or little to do with the pregnancy. So I gave Celia a cheat sheet of questions to ask Dr. K. and hoped for the best. I would meet him in a month, at which point, we would schedule the level-two ultrasound and I could see how Celia and the baby were faring. During those interim weeks friends and family would ask about the pregnancy, but I had no information to share. All I knew was that Celia felt well, which might have been an adequate response to most people, but not to me. After years of vigilant observation of and attention to every facet of conception and pregnancy, I felt alienated and disengaged from something about which I cared and had invested so much.

After four weeks of what I felt was insufficient communication between Celia and me, I flew to L.A. for Celia's seventeen week appointment with Dr. K.. Entering Dr. K.'s office, which occupied the first floor of a blue and white Victorian house, was like being transported through a time machine. All of the walls of the different rooms of his practice were covered with nineteenth-century style flowered wallpaper. The dusky pink and blue upholstered chairs in the waiting room that had probably once been a parlor, seemed to be remnants of the 1970's and paradoxically fit in only in that they too were anachronistic. Even the equipment in the exam rooms didn't look up-to-date. Dr. K. was no exception. He was rather aged, and his manner was that of an old-fashioned small town doctor, who I didn't think still existed. He was exceedingly friendly to Celia and me. I went out of my way to be affable and enthusiastic, knowing that he had had little experience working with surrogates and sensing that he wasn't a strong proponent of surrogacy. Dr. K . told me repeatedly about couples he had helped to adopt children and kept using the word "blessed" when describing those families. The word "blessed," not often used by doctors, made me nervous. I suspect that he is a religious Christian who disapproved of many reproductive technologies. Was this his way of chastising me? Was he implying that he could help us adopt a child in the future? I found his comments and manner quite unnerving, but was comforted by the fact that he performed a standard pregnancy exam, was thorough, seemed competent, and asked Celia the usual questions about the state of her pregnancy. He also recommended that we schedule the level-two ultrasound. At least he used twentieth-century technologies, if not those of the twenty-first. I kept reminding myself that given his age and long-standing affiliation with a legitimate hospital, he had probably delivered thousands of babies.

Dr. K.'s nurse, sporting a beehive and pastel print nursing outfit, added yet another era to the house of anachronisms. She too was cloyingly friendly and spoke to Celia and me as if we were young children. I suppose I was grateful that she explained the purposes of the blood tests to the fairly clueless Celia, but I was not interested in being patronized by Miss 1950's, who treated me as if I knew nothing and were merely a friend accompanying Celia to her check up. But there was nothing I could say or do but smile and nod. Marsha had warned me that Celia's obstetrician would treat her as the patient. I'd have to deal with or be condescended to by Dr. K. only a few more times. I just had to muster up the energy to behave myself and continue smiling at him.

The level-two ultrasound was scheduled for week twenty-two of the pregnancy. It would be performed by another doctor who used the facilities in Dr. K's office. It was hard to imagine that his practice possessed such advanced capabilities. During the intervening weeks, I called Celia regularly, and as always, she returned my calls at her leisure. According to her, she felt fine and the pregnancy was going smoothly. During one phone discussion at the start of the twentieth week, she casually mentioned that the baby had been kicking. While I didn't expect her to call me in the middle of the night to inform me, I did want her to share, in a timely manner, her pregnancy experiences of carrying Roger's and my baby. More and more, I suspected that she was doing this primarily for the money and didn't want to be particularly inconvenienced. We also hadn't heard from Marsha in close to two months. She finally left a message, while Roger and I were out, saying that she was just checking in and that she would be out of town at a conference and unavailable for the next week. In my imagined exit interview with the surrogacy agency I would have said that Marsha and Celia were basically competent but needed to extend themselves more and show more enthusiasm for their jobs.

When week twenty-two of the pregnancy finally arrived, Roger and I flew to L.A. for the ultrasound. Although this same test had ultimately failed to accurately predict the outcomes of my own pregnancies, I still viewed the ultrasound as a sort of green light; if everything looked okay, the pregnancy would proceed smoothly. Roger and I met Celia at her house and then walked over to Dr. K.'s strangely timeless office, which proved highly amusing to Roger. The doctor who performed the ultrasound was a spunky, no-nonsense blonde, whose style suggested 1980's suburban Southern California, adding yet another era to the mix. She seemed competent, efficient, and thorough. The ultrasound showed that we would be having a healthy baby girl whose organs were developing properly and who was right on target for her gestational age. We were delighted, and relieved, and dazed all at once. While we knew that this pregnancy was likely to have a positive outcome, we still lacked complete faith. So Roger and I, all aflutter, and Celia, casual and calm as always, went out to lunch and discussed baby names and room décor. The next few weeks went by in the same manner to which I had not become accustomed: no word from Marsha, insufficient contact and uninformative chats with Celia, and a mix of hope and fear on my part.

Although the state of the pregnancy and health of the baby were always on my mind, to some degree, the middle months of the pregnancy were fairly boring. I suppose that in this case, no news was good news or dull was preferable to the type of excitement I had undergone. Since Celia was not particularly forthcoming, I missed out on colorful anecdotes about her pregnancy experiences; doctor appointments at this point were pretty undramatic—just routine tests and no fancy ultrasounds. Basically, until the last few weeks of the pregnancy, before I dared to believe that we were really having a baby and it was safe to purchase supplies, I waited and wondered.

For me, week thirty-two of the pregnancy was a turning point. For the first time I felt optimistic that we would actually have a live, healthy baby. If Celia had gone into labor at that point, the baby would likely have been alright. I gave my friends permission to throw me the long-delayed baby shower. I ordered a car seat, stroller, and crib and tentatively bought some baby outfits. I pored through the numerous books and manuals we had acquired over the years about baby care and development, and we enrolled in a class on infant care. Roger and I began to tell more casual acquaintances and colleagues that we were expecting, and we finally chose a name for our baby, which was a topic we had nervously avoided as if such confidence about her arrival would jinx the pregnancy or that the act of naming would not make it so.

When I accompanied Celia to her doctor's appointment at thirty-four weeks, I felt even more hopeful. Celia's protruding big round belly reassured me, as did the baby's strong heartbeat and Dr. K.'s and the nurse's delight about Celia's health. The doctor observed that the baby was breech. There was still time for her to flip over, he reassured Celia, so he wasn't overly concerned, but he recommended that Celia have an ultrasound on her next visit and noted that this situation raised the possibility of a C-section. Celia, who had had three normal vaginal deliveries was not particularly pleased about the prospect of a C-section but seemed to take it in stride as she did most things. After the check up, Celia and I visited the hospital to get a lay of the land, pre-register, and explain our situation. Although we were both disappointed to discover that only two people could remain with Celia in the labor and delivery room, meaning her mother and me and excluding Roger and Miguel, I was satisfied with the hospital facilities and staff and was reassured, again, that this might really work.

Evidently, Celia was more upset about the mere possibility of having a C-section than she let on, or Marsha was meddling inappropriately, because the day after I returned home I received a message from the long-absent Marsha about Celia's concern about the C-section and a request that we provide Celia with housekeeping help for the last few weeks of the pregnancy. While I was more than happy to cover the costs of any additional household help that Celia wanted or needed, I resented Marsha's sudden phone call after months of ignoring both Celia and me, and I was annoyed by her tone and implication that we were somehow negligent of our poor, suffering surrogate. Celia, with whom I had just spent the previous day, never mentioned feeling overwhelmed by housework or overly fatigued. In fact, I was pleasantly surprised by how gracefully and comfortably she carried herself and noted that she continued to run errands and participate in family and social events. I couldn't help but wonder if Marsha brought up the topic with Celia and then presented the situation to me as if it was Celia's complaint. Simply, by the manner in which she recounted her discussion with Celia and in the way that she phrased her request, Marsha created a problem where none existed and provoked anxiety when I was finally feeling calmer and hopeful.

When I called Celia a few days later she continued to express her anxieties about having a C-section. Her belief in the omnipotence of her body had been unsettled, and like Donna, she would have to accept that not every pregnancy is identical and may present various surprises. Besides assuaging her by emphasizing that it was by no means certain that she'd even require a C-section and trying to focus on the few benefits of a C-section, such as knowing the delivery date and avoiding labor pain, I also had to respond calmly and rationally to Celia's less reasonable concerns about C-sections. For instance, despite the fact that she is Catholic, she had decided that she would try to get pregnant again to have another child of her own three months after our baby was born because, according to some Buddhist calendar, June would be an auspicious month for her to conceive a baby. She then worried that a C-section might delay her ability to get pregnant in June, the month designated by a religion that Celia does not practice. She also obsessed about the scar left from the C-section, which I reassured her wouldn't be that big since the surgery would be planned and would be low down on her abdomen and would fade in time. She then declared, what was proving to be the surrogate motto, that "everything happens for a reason" but couldn't understand the reason she'd have to have a C-section that would leave a scar. It's a good thing that this conversation took place via telephone so that she could not see me seething. Did she remember who she was talking to? What reason was there for my losing two babies? What reason was there for undergoing numerous failed rounds of IVF? How extraordinary that she could accept God's great plan for what I had senselessly undergone but found it difficult to accept that she MIGHT have a scar and a few weeks of discomfort for something that she willingly undertook knowing the risks that come with any pregnancy. I certainly wanted her to have a smooth, problem-free delivery but was taken aback by her complaining to me of all people. And so much for Marsha, whose job it was to help Celia. She clearly did little to calm her concerns and she never returned my call. I expected to hear from her next only when she was fomenting a new problem.

Despite my best efforts to smooth over differences and desire to pretend that the problem didn't exist or that I could somehow overcome it, I found it difficult to ignore the significant class and educational differences first between Donna and me and now Celia and me. From the onset of our surrogacy experiences I was concerned about working so intimately with someone with whom I had so little in common. With the exception of surrogacy arrangements in which a family member or close friend carries the baby, most surrogacy relationships entail a younger, lower-class, less-educated woman being paid to carry the baby of an older, wealthier, better-educated woman. For the most part, I could rationalize that Donna and Celia volunteered to be surrogates, and chose to help Roger and me. We treated each other as friends and were kind and pleasant to one another. However, despite both surrogates' insistence that they were not working for money and mostly wanted to help a couple have a child, they were being paid for their labors or services. In a sense, we were their employers but pretended that we were receiving a favor gratis. I never got the sense that Donna felt patronized by Roger and me or noticed any significant class differences. I believe that she viewed us as genuine, long-term friends, no different than her other close acquaintances. Celia was harder to read. I don't know that she observed meaningful differences between us, but she seemed to be more aware of the financial and contractual basis of our relationship. I suspect that I will never be entirely comfortable with the class-related aspects of surrogacy. It touched too closely to using a wet nurse or to the Biblical tale of the problematic relationship of Sarah and Hagar and its complicated aftermath. In the modern-day version, friendship and personal sacrifice were too intertwined with money and contracts, which tarnished the whole relationship. I was in the paradoxical position of patron and supplicant or benefactor and recipient. This business partnership or pseudo-friendship was further complicated by my subtle, lingering resentment that someone other than me, whom I didn't even really know that well, but to whom I was deeply grateful, was carrying my baby.

Much to everyone's surprise and delight, Dr. K. determined at the next appointment that the baby had in fact flipped downwards, meaning that a C-section would not be necessary. Celia later mentioned to me that she thought she felt significant movement a few days earlier but wasn't sure if the baby was turning or just wiggling around. Again, it would have been nice had she been more forthcoming and attentive. At this point I was just hoping that she'd have the sense to call me as soon as her water broke or labor pains began and not a few hours after she had checked into the hospital. I kept telling myself that I'd only have to deal with Celia and her doctor, frequent trips to southern California, inane conversations, and lots of forced smiling and nodding for a few more weeks.

The following weekend Roger and I attended an infant care class sponsored by our local hospital. For weeks I had been dreading sitting in a classroom populated exclusively by large-bellied women and their partners. Although I knew that no one would say anything about the fact that I wasn't pregnant, I couldn't bear the quizzical stares. The instructor began by asking everyone to introduce themselves and their due dates. I must have turned ashen at the thought and looked at Roger, for he mercifully intervened, made the introductions, and explained that we were using a surrogate. No one uttered a word or responded in any critical way, and the class proceeded normally. I was perfectly comfortable discussing our pregnancy travails and surrogacy with close friends and was even managing, after taking a deep breath, to talk about it to more casual acquaintances, but I still froze when confronted by a roomful of strangers. Perhaps people were more generous or sympathetic than I had assumed or were now better informed about surrogacy than I had been a few years earlier. In any case, I, as overly sensitive as I had become, was grateful to be spared rude comments and judgments particularly from those who had had it easy.

By the time that week thirty-eight arrived, I had begun to believe again that women, or at least some women like Celia, could walk around and conduct their daily business without triggering labor. In fact, after examining Celia, Dr. K. predicted that it seemed highly improbably that she would deliver before the due date. For the first time in five years I could focus on worrying about the delivery and health of the baby, like most mothers-to-be, instead of on premature labor. Unlike with my own two pregnancies, this time I was ready for the arrival of a newborn; my bags were packed, the baby's room was set up, and we were well-supplied with all manner of necessary and not-so-necessary infant-care equipment. At this point, I was just waiting for the call.

Since Dr. K. was confident that our baby would not be arriving early or even by the official due date, Roger and I, reluctantly, waited until three days before the official birth date to drive to Los Angeles. We nervously and guiltily felt that we were cutting it close by arriving in L.A. on Saturday when the baby was due on Monday, but were reassured by the doctor that there was no rush. On Monday, March 12, the due date, nothing happened. The next day we accompanied Celia to her appointment with Dr. K., who declared that Celia was in no way ready to deliver and that barring any changes, which he found highly unlikely, he would not induce for another week. So Roger and I, cell phones in hand, tried to distract ourselves and enjoy L.A. for at least a week. We ate well, attended a play, a concert, visited museums, and drove around but were always on edge waiting for our cell phones to ring. We called Celia daily, who, amused by our nervousness, reassured us that she felt fine and was not in labor. Family and friends called often wanting updates; every ring of the phone made us jump and having to reassure others that all was well and that nothing was happening only wound us up more. One Sunday morning I practically jumped out of my skin when my phone rang at six o'clock a.m. only to be disappointed to hear, oddly enough, from a priest, Father McGarrity in San Francisco, who had mistakenly dialed my number. Our stay in L.A. was surreal. We lived in a hotel, not knowing exactly when we'd be checking out and feeling removed from what was familiar and comforting. How utterly ironic and ridiculous that the baby, who I feared above all else would arrive too early, would now come late.

One week after the due date and nine nail-biting days in Los Angeles we joined Celia, yet again, at Dr. K's, who once more declared that Celia didn't appear to be making any progress on the labor and delivery front. However, he agreed to begin inducing her that evening and expected her to deliver some time late the next day. Roger and I were planning to move to a hotel closer to the hospital, but Dr. K. assured us that there was no rush. We should get a good night sleep in L.A. and come to the hospital in the late morning or early afternoon. Celia would be in touch with us. That evening Celia checked into the hospital while Roger and I tried futilely to remain calm. We talked with her that evening, and she reported that she felt fine and was planning to go to sleep early and would call us in the morning.

The next morning at six o'clock, Celia, less calm and collected than usual, called to tell me that she was six centimeters dilated and in labor and that Roger and I should come to the hospital as soon as possible. Apparently, she responded more quickly to the inducement than Dr. K. has anticipated. We quickly dressed and packed and drove to the hospital which was about thirty minutes away. After checking in and being told that we would have our own room in which we could stay with our baby until she was ready to go home with us, we were taken to Celia's delivery room. Much to our delight, Roger was told that he would be allowed to stay in Celia's room for the delivery along with me and Celia's mother. Celia seemed tired but cheerful and excited. Her mother, who lived nearby, had already made herself at home and was helping Celia to breathe through her contractions and relax. Shortly after we had arrived a nurse came in to examine Celia and then called in Dr. K. who declared that Celia was ready to deliver and should begin pushing soon. Various nurses and doctors were summoned, Celia's mother stood behind her to help her push, and Roger and I were told to stand near the head of Celia's bed so that we could see the baby emerge but still allow Celia some space and dignity. In what was record time for Celia and what even seemed speedy to me, a mere two hours after we arrived at the hospital, our baby daughter Anna was born. She weighed nine pounds, was twenty-one inches long, and was a healthy, hearty, screaming redhead. After nine days of waiting in Los Angeles, which had been preceded by five years of waiting and trying to have a baby, perfect Anna arrived quickly and relatively smoothly; and we barely made it on time for her long-awaited entry into this world.

Oddly enough, the birth experience and our time in the hospital were not weird. Although Celia delivered Anna, Roger and I were treated as her parents and felt like her parents. After the doctor and nurses, we were the first to hold her, feed her, and watch the nurse give Anna her first bath. All of the hospital staff we met congratulated Roger and me on our new daughter and treated me as Anna's mother. I was astonished by the kindness and professionalism of everyone at the hospital as if they encountered surrogacy arrangements all the time.

After Roger and I had a chance to spend some time with our baby girl and Celia got some rest, we went to visit her in her room down the hall from us and introduce her to Anna. Again, I was surprised by how normal it seemed to meet her extended family and have Celia hold Anna. I didn't feel threatened or uncomfortable while our baby was in Celia's arms. Her family was warm and supportive and behaved as though they too viewed surrogacy as a commonplace event. Perhaps since Celia had done this before it was to them; nonetheless, they appeared to be genuinely pleased about Anna's arrival and Celia's good deed.

Two days later, a day after Celia was discharged from the hospital, we drove home with our healthy baby daughter. The journey home was easy and problem free, much like Anna's birth. In comparison to every other birth and pregnancy-related experience I'd undergone, Anna's birth, was lacking in high drama. Although the event was exciting, joyous, and long-awaited, it was typical in the sense that it was absolutely standard and basically according to plan. For the first time in many years of attempted pregnancies and deliveries we did not experience, disappointment, failure, illness, serious complications, or loss. What was unusual or dramatic for Roger and me was the normalcy of Anna's birth. Like any new parents we would now have to adjust to a new life with a baby, but unlike many first-time parents, we took nothing for granted. I would also need to learn to assume the best and accept that perhaps pregnancy and birth are not pathologies and that newborns can be robust and healthy. Most importantly, I would need to work on dissolving the sadness, anxiety, pain, and sense of failure that had built up over the previous five years so that I would not "shed" "more tears over answered prayers than unanswered ones" (St. Teresa) and instead, like most parents, rejoice in the birth and life of our new daughter.

## About the Author

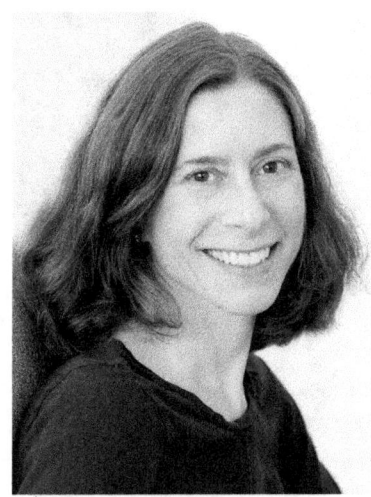

Author photo by Hope Hudson

Ariel Balter earned a BA in psychology from Bryn Mawr College and an MA and PhD in English from Tufts University. Over the past fifteen years she has taught English and writing at various universities, colleges, and high schools, presented papers at academic conferences, and published several academic essays, including an article on Edith Wharton and one on James Weldon Johnson. *The Maternity Labyrinth* is her first work of creative nonfiction. She is currently working on a novel.

Ariel Balter lives in California with her husband and daughter.

www.ingramcontent.com/pod-product-compliance
Lightning Source LLC
Chambersburg PA
CBHW052103070526
44584CB00017B/2307